Published by Sterling & Ross Publishers
New York, NY 10001
www.SterlingandRoss.com

Cover design by Brian Goff
Composition/typography by Polina Bartashnik
Cover photography © Nederpelt Media Corp. 2006,
All Rights Reserved.

10 9 8 7 6 5 4 3 2

Printed in the United States of America.

THE BIRD-FLU PRIMER

The Guide to Being Prepared and Surviving an Avian Flu Pandemic

Larry Altshuler, M.D.

NEW YORK   TORONTO   LONDON

TABLE OF CONTENTS

➤ INTRODUCTION

"This bird flu is going to demolish the economy and screw up civilization as we know it," said one Internet post in early 2006. While these words may not become reality, the worldwide spread of a lethal virus has the potential for devastating consequences. Many Americans are watching the media for any updates on what is known as the avian (bird) flu, as cases are reported across the globe. The majority of people feel they

> *"The Bird-Flu is going to demolish the economy and screw-up civilization as we know it."*
> -2006 Internet post.

are helpless to do anything about a possible pandemic and have simply resigned themselves to relying on the government and public health agencies to protect them and their families. As we saw with the abysmal Federal, State and local reaction to a hurricane which killed almost 1500 Americans in 2005, the possibility of any meaningful assistance coming from those same agencies when dealing with a disease outbreak that could kill millions, is remote at best. With that prospect in mind, Americans and citizens of the world need to arm themselves for what might be a deadly viral war the likes of which has not been seen in almost one hundred years. That being said, with the right information and guidance, YOU can be ready to deal with events that your government and public health officials will not, or cannot, deal with.

Now, that may seem daunting, considering you're unlikely to be an expert on internal medicine or infectious disease. But one thing to remember is that, if and when a bird flu pandemic hits your area, many experts agree that the time frame of devastation will last from as little as several weeks to an outside of 18 months. As a result, if you can keep yourself and your family safe for this period of time, you'll be out of the woods—we'll all be out of the woods. Unfortunately, those who don't take the necessary precautions (medicinal, societal, and familial) are risking not only their lives and the lives of their loved ones, but the possible happiness and prosperity of generations to come.

THE BIRD FLU PRIMER is your one-stop-shop for all things related to the avian flu. No other book tells you what you can do to prepare for an outbreak, medically (conventional and alternative), as well as what to do strategically if a bird flu pandemic does strike. We offer several expert-derived scenarios to help you recognize the stages in which we might find ourselves and where we might end up.

In addition to this value-added advice, THE BIRD FLU PRIMER includes everything you need to know about the actual disease—how it affects animals and humans, how it kills, and what methods are currently available and being developed to fight the virus, as well as their chances for success. Perhaps most importantly this book will show you specific steps to prevent the contraction of the potentially deadly virus—after all, it is fatal for over 50% of those who contract it. These steps include lessons from the pandemic of 1918 and how H5N1 (the deadly bird flu virus) is similar and how it differs from that benchmark outbreak.

THE BIRD FLU PRIMER also includes expert opinion from all sides of the debate, from those who believe this is nothing but fear-mongering to those experts who are absolutely certain the bird flu pandemic is nearly upon us. With reasoned guidance and medical fact I will show you and your family what to be concerned with and what to dismiss. We'll separate fact from fiction (and address some issues not covered in the traditional media) as we navigate the potentially deadly waters of a pandemic not seen in our lifetimes. Despite most people's fears, this disease can be defeated, but knowledge is currently the only antidote.

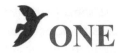

ONE

BIRD FLU: WHAT IT IS AND WHY YOU NEED TO KNOW ABOUT IT

We've all had the flu, most of us many times during our lives. When we do, the symptoms are miserable; you feel awful, your head pounds, your muscles and joints ache, your nose drips, you have little or no energy. Sometimes, you feel like you're going to die.

Fortunately, most of us recover from the flu. Some however, do not. If you're very young or very old, or have certain chronic diseases, you can die from the everyday strain of influenza (the flu). In fact, about 36,000 Americans die of the flu every year. If you are healthy, however, you should recover, unless the flu virus is extremely powerful. Then, everyone, including healthy people, has a higher risk of dying. The bird flu is one of those strains that can become that powerful...and that deadly.

The bird flu is exactly that- a flu virus that originates in birds. This virus is usually only transmitted among bird species, but in specific circumstances (which I will explain shortly), it can be transmitted from birds to humans. And in even more specific cases, it can be transmitted from human to human. Such a virus can become virulent; that is, it can break down your protective mechanisms and wreak havoc on your body. The more virulent it is, the more damage- and death- it can cause.

The present bird flu, called H5N1, is already a virulent strain. When tested in chick embryos, all died. Half of the humans infected have died. The H5N1 virus has the potential to change, or mutate, and gain the ability to easily spread to and among humans, which is why scientists are so concerned. If it doesn't, that's great. If it does however, it will occur rapidly and will be devastating. The H5N1 strain may be around for a long time, and the longer it is, the greater the possibility it will mutate and spread through humans.

A consultant to institutional investors and biotech companies regarding the avian flu, Rich Macary, says, "Indonesia almost made the call to go to Pandemic Phase 4 recently. They were within 24 hours of calling it Human to Human and raising the threat level. In Indonesia, people are getting bird flu who have no business getting bird flu, who don't work around poultry- an accountant, a government worker. There are plenty of signs that human to human contact is occurring. In fact, the World Health Organization (WHO) released a paper that said some of these clusters looked human to human—though at this point it's all circumstantial—that is, it's hard to prove whether it is or it isn't." (See more about different levels of pandemics in Chapter 2).

You should also be aware that whether this particular virus spreads and becomes lethal or not, most scientists agree that sooner or later, some viral strain will become powerful and lethal. It is only a matter of time. According to Dr. Jeffrey Taubenberger of the Armed Forces Institute of Pathology (AFIP), "I think pandemics are practically inevitable, but not necessarily H5N1." Even if the current H5N1 strain fades away in a few years, it could return. In fact, as you can see in Figure A, three previous bird flu strains have reappeared decades after their initial appearance. Two of these (H2N2 and H3N2) became more destructive and caused epidemics when they reappeared. So, the only thing that you can do is to be prepared.

CRYING WOLF?

Many authorities and authors are dismissing fears of the bird flu virus, saying that we have nothing to worry about in terms of the occurence of a pandemic. Other authorities say the opposite. In fact, our government is currently stockpiling medications for a possible pandemic and preparing plans for exactly that.

Should you worry? After all, as you will read below, there have been other bird flu viruses which have not ended up being much more serious than seasonal flu viruses. Each time, fears have been raised about a possible severe pandemic, but it never occurred. The same may happen with the H5N1 bird flu virus. It may fade away totally or change into a virus that causes only mild disease. On the other hand, there is always a possibility it will become a virulent virus that spreads quickly throughout the world, wreaking havoc on mankind. Which is the most likely scenario? No one knows, that's the scary part.

New viruses and infectious agents are being discovered yearly and these entities have been unknown or unrecognized until this century. For example, there is the prion that causes mad cow disease. Prion is short for proteinaceous infectious particle, which is made only of protein. Prions are able to convert normal molecules of the host into an abnormal structure and thus disrupt normal brain function. Another example is HIV, which suddenly appeared several decades ago and became virulent. We do not know what the future holds in terms of new infectious agents.

While there is no need for panic, there is need for awareness and preparedness. If the virus just kills birds, we can be less concerned. But if the avian flu becomes a serious threat to humans, being armed with basic knowledge of the disease will be your best survival tool.

BIRD FLU: IT HAS HAPPENED BEFORE
AND IT WILL HAPPEN AGAIN

Every few decades, a particularly virulent strain of bird flu appears and spreads rapidly throughout the world, creating what is called a pandemic. The worst pandemic in history was in 1918 and killed at least 20 to 50 million people. The exact number is unknown because most countries were unable to keep an accurate accounting. (For a more in-depth discussion about other bird-flu pandemics, see Chapter 4). There was also one in 1958, that killed 2 million, and again in 1968 that killed 700,000. Certainly, these two pandemics killed only a fraction of those killed during the1918 pandemic, which is why they haven't made the news as much, and they killed primarily the young, the old and the weak, as do the more common flu viruses. But the 1918 flu virus struck down healthy, young adults…and many millions of them.

> "Most scientists agree that sooner or later, some viral strain will become powerful and lethal. It is only a matter of time."

Several different strains of bird flu have been found in humans since 1997, and fortunately these have been limited. But as you will see, it only takes a few changes to make such a virus more lethal. TABLE 1 lists the confirmed instances of bird flu viruses infecting humans since 1997.

TABLE 1:
BIRD FLU INFECTIONS
DOCUMENTED SINCE 1997

H5N1 (same strain as current bird flu): Hong Kong, 1997. A virulent strain infected 18 people, 6 of whom died.

H9N2, China and Hong Kong, 1999. A less virulent strain infected 2 children, who both recovered.

H7N2, Virginia, 2002. A less virulent strain infected one person.

H5N1 (same strain as current), China and Hong Kong, 2003. Two cases documented in one family, with one member dying. Virulent strain.

H7N7, Netherlands, 2003. Eighty-nine people infected from poultry, with 3 human to human transmissions. Only 1 person died and the virus disappeared.

H9N2, Hong Kong, 2003. Low virulence strain infected one child, who recovered.

H7N2, New York, 2003. One hospitalized patient found to have flu virus, recovered.

H7N3, Canada, 2004. Numerous human infections in poultry workers, who primarily suffered eye infections.

H5N2, Texas, 2004. Birds on one farm were found to contain this virus. There was no transmission to humans and was contained.

H5N1 (current strain), Thailand and Vietnam, 2004, and other Asian outbreaks in 2005. Discussed above.

H5N1 (current strain), Iraq, January, 2006. Eight people hospitalized, one girl died. Still being investigated.

H5N1 (current strain), Nigeria, February 2006.First known outbreak in Africa. 40,000 out of 46,000 birds died of bird flu. No human transmission noted yet.

H5N1 (current strain), Azerbaijian, February, 2006. Annnounced outbreak of H5N1 in fowl. The strain was found in ducks and swans.

H5N1 (current strain); China, Indonesia, February 2006. Another death in Indonesia, raising the human death toll in that country to 17. Another death in China, raising its human death toll to 8. This death was in an area with no reported outbreaks in poultry.

See THE BIRD FLU PRIMER website for an updated listing as well as other expert guidance and advice at
www.TheBirdFluPrimer.com

FIGURE A:
HISTORY OF BIRD INFLUENZA

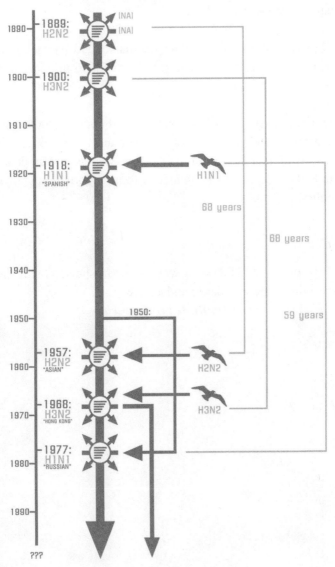

THE FLU: WHAT IS IT AND HOW DOES IT WORK?

To begin with, there are three types of flu virus, called Influenza A, Influenza B, and Influenza C. Only Influenza A viruses become virulent, or destructive, and cause pandemics, so it will be the one we'll focus on in this book. Influenza A viruses actually originate in birds, who have the greatest number and range of influenza viruses. These viral strains can occasionally cross over into mammals, primarily pigs and humans.

A virus is a small, spherical particle, about a millionth of an inch in diameter. Unlike bacteria, it is not a full cell, and cannot reproduce on its own. This is beneficial since if we can prevent it from getting into our body, it can't reproduce and cause harm. But if it does get into our body, it can use our own cells to reproduce and cause illness.

The surface of this particle is covered with spike-like projections made of protein, called hemagglutinin (we'll call them H-spikes), as well as mushroom-appearing projections also made of protein called neuraminidase (N-spikes). The purpose of these projections is to help the particle stick to the surface of cells in your respiratory tract so that the virus can then invade the cell and reproduce. It works in a similar fashion to Velcro, using tiny little hooks to hold onto receptors on the surface of cells. These proteins also help the virus invade the cell.

As I've said, because the virus particle is not a fully functioning unit, it must infect a cell to reproduce. It works much like a parasite, such as mistletoe. This plant must attach to trees to live because it uses the tree's nutrients to survive. Put mistletoe in water and it will die because it can't support itself alone. The virus particle must use the mechanisms found in human cells to support itself. Without those, it can't survive and reproduce.

Each major virus family has a different combination of these projections. In all, there are 16 subtypes of hemagglutinin and 9 subtypes of neuraminidase. Because the combinations of those subtypes vary, we are able to identify which virus family has caused infection. The current bird flu is referred to as H5N1 (Hemagglutinin 5, Neuraminidase 1). Others are notated depending on what they contain (see Table 1). Primarily, the H5 and H7 subtypes are known to cause high virulence, which is why the present virus is a cause for concern.

Inside these virus particles are segments of genes. Genes are the components that control all the functions of an organism. A flu particle contains fragments of eight genes, each fragment controlling an exact function. So, one specific gene segment directs the development of the projections on the surface while another may help the virus infect a cell and another may blunt a counter attack from the host immune system. Some genes are responsible for how virulent the flu particle can become. Based on the specific combination of these genes, some viruses may not cause problems while others can cause significant damage. So, for example, an H3N5 virus (which is the type usually seen in seasonal flu) is not as destructive as an H5N1 strain.

How do these genes control the actions of the viral particle? Within these genes are strands of material called DNA and RNA, which represent the blueprint of an organism. In other words, every organism contains their own DNA and RNA, which determines what the organism is and how each and every cell functions. Each species has different DNA and RNA, which is why every species is different. In humans, DNA is the primary controlling force, and RNA serves as a messenger for DNA, traveling around the body and initiating body functions on command from the DNA. In viruses, however, which are not as complicated as humans, RNA is the primary controlling force.

The reason this is important is because DNA and RNA are composed differently. DNA has two strands that are intertwined and RNA has only one strand. The significance is that RNA is much more prone to change. Such a change is referred to as a "mutation," and when this occurs, the messages and actions of the organism change with it.

MUTATIONS: HOW THE VIRUS CHANGES

As mentioned above, Influenza A viruses originate from birds and most often do not infect humans. To do so, they must somehow undergo a change. This change is called a mutation, which occurs in the genes of the virus. When the genes mutate, it results in the formation of different hemagglutinin and neuraminidase projections. When this occurs, it changes how the virus spreads, how it attaches to cells, and how it breaks into and infects the cell. If an Influenza A bird flu virus doesn't change, it is unable to attach or infect a human cell. But if the projections change, it then can attach/infect the human cell.

There are two types of mutations that occur. The first is called an antigenic *drift*, which occurs every few years, but involves only minor changes. This occurs when a virus gradually adapts to humans. The second is called an antigenic *shift*, in which totally new and different hemagglutinin and neuraminidase proteins suddenly occur (also referred to as "re-assortment.") When this happens, a major new pandemic virus can appear in humans. Since the year 1900, this has occurred four times, varying between one to three decades between outbreaks.

The pandemic virus strains of 1957 and 1968 occurred from an antigenic shift. The 1918 pandemic appears to have resulted from an antigenic drift. Both types of mutation are possible with the H5N1 strain.

Mutation can be beneficial or it can be dangerous. First, a mutation can make a seemingly benign virus into a virulent one. In the case of bird flu, human to human transmission is very rare at present, but a mutation can quickly change this. If it does, the virus can spread quickly throughout the world and cause significant illness and death.

A virus can also mutate several times and become stronger so it may infect people, then "hibernate" for a while, then reappear even stronger. In many cases, as it spreads and infects, it can continue to make itself stronger with additional mutations.

The other problem with mutation is that what we use to kill the virus today may not work tomorrow. The problem is that a virus is so easily adaptable, it can inherently evolve to defend itself against current antidotes or inoculations. We have seen many bacteria become resistant to antibiotics, and many flu viruses have now become resistant to antiviral medications.

Again, in the case of bird flu, any medication created to kill it may become resistant if further mutations occur. As a result, many experts believe that the antiviral drug, Tamiflu, would not save many lives and certainly not prevent a pandemic if the virus develops resistance against it.

One good aspect of mutation is that it can change a virulent virus to a more benign one. So, eventually it can disappear or become weaker, but unfortunately it might do a lot of damage and kill millions of people before it does.

It is important to know that scientists do not fully understand how viruses invade cells and what makes some viruses benign and others virulent. It is a complicated process and one that may take decades to unravel.

FIGURE B:
FLU PARTICLE

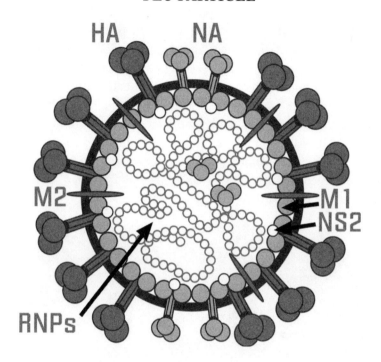

HA = Hemagglutinin
NA = Neuraminidase
RNP = RNA and nuclear material
M = Matrix protein

HOW BIRD FLU IS SPREAD TO HUMANS

Most bird flus are contained within the species of birds because the flu particle can only attach to cells in that species. If certain mutations occur, however, these virus particles can attach to human cells and cause direct damage to them. The current bird flu can do just that.

The majority of people who have been infected with H5N1 have had direct contact with infected poultry or surfaces contaminated with their feces and other secretions. The reason most cases have occurred in Asia is because many households keep small poultry flocks to eat and sell, and these chickens roam freely, entering homes and sharing outdoor areas where children play and adults work. The same is true for developing nations. Humans can also be infected by direct contact when they slaughter, de-feather, butcher or prepare infected fowl and come into contact with the insides of the birds, which may also contain the viral particles.

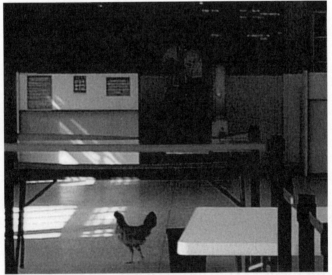

A chicken roaming freely inside an airport in the Virgin Islands.

The majority of human cases have resulted from this type of direct contact. However, there have been a few rare cases of human to human transmission. This may have occurred due to contact with overwhelming numbers of virus particles, since caregivers were the ones who were infected by other humans.

However, this doesn't mean that the virus has mutated into a form that is *easily* transmissable between humans. This would occur when the bird virus infects a human, who concurrently has been infected with another human virus. As mentioned above, what occurs is an exchange and a re-shuffling of genes between these two viruses (antigenic shift), and this mutated virus can then be transmitted between humans.

On two occasions so far, H5N1 has mixed with other viruses that have had the potential to increase the virus' ability to attach to human receptors. In October 2005, H5N1 was brought to the Middle East by migratory birds, where another avian influenza, H9N2, was present in the wild bird population. Testing of several cases in Turkey revealed that some genetic information was transferred from H9N2 to H5N1. Now that the H5N1 virus has spread to Europe, it may recombine with a swine flu virus, H1N1, which contains genes that increase the ability of the virus to attach to human receptors.

Neither of these occurrences has resulted in sustained human to human transmission, but the longer this virus spreads among chickens and other birds, the greater the possibility that a re-shuffling will occur. This is what concerns the authorities. As Dr. Anthony Fauci of the National Institute of Allergy and Infectious Disease says, "The longer you see the virus among chickens, the greater chance you get of an occasional human getting infected. And when an occasional human gets infected, if the human is also infected with a human flu virus, there is the possibility of a recombination of genes to get a virus that more efficiently spreads from human to human."

HOW THE FLU VIRUS HARMS US AND HOW WE DEFEND OURSELVES

To infect a human and produce damage, a flu particle must get inside the human cell, which then allows it to replicate. When it does get inside the human cell, it basically interferes with the normal processes of that cell so that it cannot work properly. In the meantime, it uses the cell's structure and processes for its own benefit, especially replicating and spreading to other cells. Thus the damage spreads.

Many flu particles have their own ability to split cells, enter the cells and then replicate themselves. Although much of the mechanism is still unknown, it is recognized that the hemmaglutinin and neuraminidase proteins on the surface of the cell can both contribute to the activation of the flu particle. Often, however, the host cell and immune system can produce enzymes in response to the flu particle that actually help the virus get inside the cell.

Once the virus has the ability to infect cells and spread, damage results in many ways. For one, the virus can simply stop the functions of the cells it infects, causing the organ to malfunction or even stop working, or splitting the cell, destroying it. It does so by triggering the release of various substances, such as histamine, leukotrienes, interleukins, tumor necrosis factor, and cytokines, all which can cause harmful reactions and damage to the body. Since most viruses infect the lungs, this can lead to viral pneumonia and resultant difficulty breathing and getting oxygen into the body.

After the virus renders these cells non-functional, the damaged cells can become a breeding ground for another invader-bacteria. This is referred to as a "secondary bacterial infection," which can do even more damage than the virus does. Over half the deaths due to influenza are caused by bacterial pneumonia.

Fortunately, most viruses do not kill large numbers of humans. It is not fully understood how viruses kill some people but not others. We do know, however, that our immune system gears up when invaded by a virus, producing antibodies that bind to the hemagglutinin and neuraminidase projections, preventing further spreading and destroying the viral particle. When enough antibodies are produced, they quell the invasion and the symptoms resolve.

Our immune system is very efficient at destroying these viral invaders. Sometimes, however, it is too efficient. In many cases, especially with some bird flu viruses, the immune system overreacts, resulting in what is called Acute Respiratory Distress Syndrome (ARDS) This over-reaction is what occurred with the SARS virus (see box, page 29). In short, the immune system cells accumulate in areas of damage and release substances that can harm cells rather than protect or repair them. This may be the reason the bird flu can kill people who are otherwise healthy and have strong immune systems. So, ironically, those with weaker immune systems may be able to survive some bird flu viruses better than those with stronger immune systems.

The bird flu at this time is called pneumotropic, meaning it affects the respiratory tract. However, such viruses can mutate and become neurotropic (affecting the nervous system) or pantropic (affecting all the body systems) by spreading through the bloodstream. So, the lungs are not the only organ systems that can become involved. The virus can spread throughout the body and infect other organs, and can exacerbate chronic diseases such as diabetes, heart disease and kidney disease. When these diseases are made worse, the body is further weakened, allowing the virus to cause even more damage.

Once again, scientists do not fully understand all the mechanisms by which the flu virus exerts its damaging effects and how our own immune system may complicate matters. In fact, recent research has shown that bird viruses have a different molecular characteristic that human viruses don't have. As a result, it allows them to interact with human cells and potentially shut down pathways in those cells. Until we understand more about these mechanisms, preventing death from a virulent strain may be very difficult.

THE PRESENT BIRD FLU VIRUS: WHAT IT HAS DONE SO FAR

Bird flu normally infects only birds, both domestic and migratory. In domestic poultry, there are two main forms of the virus, characterized by low and high virulence. Low virulence forms cause only mild symptoms, such as ruffled feathers and a drop in egg production. High virulence forms spread very rapidly through flocks, affect multiple organs in the chickens, and kill almost all the chickens infected, usually within 48 hours.

Migratory birds can of course spread these viruses faster than domestic birds since the latter are more confined and their secretions are limited to specific areas. Wild waterfowl are considered to be the main carriers of Influenza A viruses and have been so for centuries. It is known that migratory birds are the ones that have passed this virus to domestic fowl. Fortunately, most of these strains are of low virulence. Rarely have high virulence viruses been found in migratory birds, but these birds have been found dead within short distances from domestic birds. However, it is thought that the H5N1 virus is being spread by migratory birds to chickens in the more virulent form.

This is disconcerting for two reasons. First, migratory birds cannot be easily secluded and therefore will continue to pass this virulent strain to fowl in other countries. This has already occurred. The H5N1 virus has been found in dead migratory birds in Africa and Europe only since the start of 2006. Second, although so far most migratory birds carrying H5N1 have died, it appears that they are still spreading the virus. This may be the result of some birds becoming carriers of the virus without becoming sick, or being able to pass on the virus before they die. Either way, this will spread the virus even faster and

THE SARS VIRUS:
SIMILARITIES AND DIFFERENCES

Many people are familiar with the SARS virus, which started in Asia in 2003 and rapidly spread throughout the world. SARS suddenly appeared in a businessman in Guangdong province in China and soon spread to four health care workers who treated him. It was the first severe and readily transmissible new disease to appear in the 21st century.

SARS infected several thousand people, with an overall death rate of 10%. There were 8,422 cases and 916 deaths, one third in Hong Kong. Ninety per-cent of people infected recovered. It was primarily noted in Hong Kong, but cases were seen throughout the world (30 countries), including Canada and the U.S. It was transmitted between humans in close contact, especially among health care workers, and did not involve widespread infection.

SARS was an epidemic, not a pandemic. An epidemic is a disease that appears as new cases in a given human population, during a given period, at a rate that substantial-ly exceeds what is expected, based on recent experience. Usually, an epidemic is relegated to one area or several scattered areas and is contained. The SARS epidemic was caused by a coronavirus, which is not as virulent or lethal as an avian virus. However, it spread very easily and when it did kill, it did so using the same mechanisms as a bird flu virus. At one point, officials were concerned that the SARS virus would become pandemic but fortunately it was contained.

more extensively.

There are other reasons for concern as well. Since mid-2003, the virus has caused large scale death in almost 200 million poultry, primarily in Asia. It is the largest and most severe in history and has never been seen in so many countries simultaneously. The virus is also very tenacious, meaning it is hard to eradicate and more resistant to treatment (see Chapter 5).

The H5N1 bird flu was thought to be totally contained by March 2004, yet by June of that same year, more outbreaks were documented, and are ongoing. In fact, in parts of Southeast Asia, especially Cambodia and Vietnam, the virus has become endemic, meaning it continues to be carried in large populations of birds. More recently, it has spread to Iraq, Nigeria, Italy, Greece and Switzerland.

This is very concerning, as confirmed by Dr. Anthony Fauci, Director of the NIAID: "The events have shown a clearcut expansion of the infection either in migratory birds or going from the migratory birds to the chicken flocks."

Of the few avian flu viruses that have infected humans, the H5N1 virus has also caused the largest number of cases of severe illness and death. Although the 1918 pandemic killed millions of people, the percentage of people killed who are infected by the H5N1 virus is much greater and those that become infected are much sicker. Most cases have occurred in previously healthy children and young adults. So far, there are believed to be just a few cases of human to human transmission, having occurred in what experts term 'family clusters'—though as previously stated, in those cases where members of the same family have died in a cluster, there has usually been symptomatic evidence that a single bird source was to blame— however some experts dispute this hypothesis.

WHERE HAS THE BIRD FLU BEEN?

POULTRY (ongoing)

Cambodia
Kazakhstan
China
Malaysia
Tibet
Mongolia
Indonesia
Russia
Japan
Iraq
Laos
Nigeria
South Korea
Vietnam
Thailand

POULTRY OUT-BREAKS (not ongoing)

Turkey
Romania
Ukraine

MIGRATORY BIRD OUTBREAKS

China
Croatia
Hong Kong
Mongolia
Romania
Azerbaijan
Greece
Italy
Romania
Bulgaria
India
Greece
Switzerland

HUMAN CASES

Cambodia
China
Indonesia
Thailand
Vietnam
Turkey

for a complete update visit
www.TheBirdFluPrimer.com

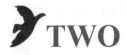

TWO

PANDEMIC

THE REASON TO WORRY: PANDEMIC

As mentioned, one risk of the bird flu is its spread from birds to humans. As long as it can only spread directly from fowl and poultry to humans, it can be contained. But the greatest risk is that the virus could mutate into a form that is highly virulent and contagious for humans and thus spreads rapidly from person to person. Stopping the virus' spread in chickens can be done by killing infected chickens. But not so with humans--- once it starts spreading, it could continue to envelope the world. If this occurs, it is called a pandemic. According to the WHO and the CDC, there are six major phases of a flu pandemic, as follows:

Interpandemic period

Phase 1: No new influenza virus subtypes have been detected in humans. An influenza virus subtype that has caused human infection may be present in animals. If present in animals, the risk of human infection or disease is considered to be low. In the case of H5N1, this would mean there are no poultry outbreaks.

Phase 2: No new influenza virus subtypes have been detected in humans. However, a circulating animal influenza virus subtype poses a substantial risk of human disease. In the case of H5N1, there are poultry cases, but no human cases.

Pandemic alert period

Phase 3: Human infection(s) with a new subtype but no human-to-human spread, or at most, rare instances of spread to a close contact. In the case of H5N1, there are human cases with clear history of exposure to chickens, but limited human-to-human transmission.

Phase 4: Small cluster(s) with limited human-to-human transmission but spread is highly localized, suggesting that the virus is not well adapted to humans. In the case of H5N1, this would occur if there were clusters of human cases, involving less than 25 cases that lasted two weeks.

Phase 5: Larger cluster(s) but human-to-human spread still localized, suggesting that the virus is becoming increasingly better adapted to humans but may not yet be fully transmissible (substantial pandemic risk). In the case of H5N1, the total number of cases is not rapidly increasing, but clusters of 25-50 people are infected over 2-4 weeks. Cases are usually localized (e.g., to a village, island, military base).

Pandemic period

Phase 6: Pandemic: increased and sustained transmission in general population. This means sustained and continued transmission with steadily increasing number of cases.

The 1918 bird flu virus was a Phase 6 pandemic. It spread throughout the world killing millions of people. The H5N1 virus may do the same, if three conditions are met:

1) A new influenza virus subtype emerges.
2) It infects humans, causing serious illness.

3) It spreads easily and sustainably among humans.

At present, the first two conditions have already been met. This equates to Phase 3, which is a pandemic alert period. Whether human-to-human transmission (Phases 4-6) develops is still unknown. But the risk that the H5N1 virus will acquire this ability will be present as long as opportunities for human infection continue. In turn, these opportunities will be present as long as the virus continues to infect birds. So, this possibility may persist for years to come.

> **"Pandemics can also occur more than once. Eventually, it can return to the same community and attack again, either with the same virulent strain or, in a worst case scenario, in a newer and more deadly strain."**

Dr. Jeffrey Taubenberger of the AFIP agrees: "The more broadly this virus circulates in domestic and wild birds in more geographic regions, the larger the cumulative risk that the virus could further adapt to humans by either mutation or re-assortment with a co-circulating strain."

It cannot be stressed enough that as long as the H5N1 virus is present and continues to spread, the higher the risk for a full blown Phase 6 pandemic. As I related previously, human transmission occurs when a virus such as the H5N1 either mutates on its own or infects a human who, at the same time, is infected with a human virus (re-assortment). The traditional seasonal flu is easily passed between humans but is not serious to all but the weakest in society—we've all had it and survived it. On the other hand, the avian flu is potentially deadly, but as long as you don't handle infected birds, you're safe. However, if these two strains come together and exchange genetic information, there exists the potential for the worst of both possible worlds—of an easily transmittable, deadly flu. As long as the H5N1 virus is present and can be transmitted to humans from fowl, this scenario can take place.

PHASE 3: A CAUSE FOR CONCERN

Should you be concerned? Yes, this is a serious threat.

According to Dr. Taubenberger, "I think the chances of human adaptation through either mutation or re-assortment are low but certainly not zero. Since the outcome is so severe, even small risk must be considered a serious threat." Chillingly he told me, "I think if H5N1 adapts to humans it will cause a bad pandemic, possibly akin to 1918."

Phase 3 is labeled as an 'alert stage,' and for good reason, as detailed above. The current virus has not disappeared or become weaker and is present in large parts of the globe. In addition, it has spread to more poultry as well as birds that migrate to new areas and can infect other migratory birds as well as other domestic fowl. All these factors increase the risk of the virus changing into one that can be transferred among humans. Once again, as the virus spreads, there is more chance it will cause a pandemic.

That's not all, however. According to the World Health Organization, several distinct characteristics are emerging with this potent and dangerous strain of bird flu virus:

1) When compared to H5N1 strains from 1997 and 2004, current H5N1 strains are more lethal when injected into mice and ferrets (which mimic humans) and survive longer.

2) The subtype (H5N1) mutates rapidly.

3) The H5N1 strain has expanded its host range, meaning it has infected and killed mammalian species that previously were resistant to infection with bird viruses.

4) It causes severe disease in humans, with a high case-fatality rate.

5) The virus has spread rapidly throughout poultry flocks in Asia, increasing the likelihood of infecting humans or pigs. In this event, genetic reassortment with human strains could occur, leading to a new pandemic strain.

6) The viral behavior in waterfowl, where it is naturally found, may be changing. In the spring of 2005, nearly 6000 migratory birds died of a highly virulent form of H5N1 in a nature preserve in China. This was considered very unusual and not seen previously. There have been two large so-called die-offs in the past; in South Africa in 1961 (H5N3 strain) and in Hong Kong in the winter of 2002-2003 (the H5N1 strain).

7) In chickens, symptoms are evident and those animals can be removed from the population, but it has been discovered that some domestic ducks can transmit the virus to other birds without showing any symptoms, which complicates control efforts and removes any warning signals for humans.

8) The virus is continuing to spread through migratory birds to other areas of the world, including Russia and Europe.

9) Recent investigation on the H5N1 strain from Turkey demonstrates that the strains contain two mutations which may make the virus better adapted to humans. These mutations could potentially enhance transmission from birds to humans and between humans.

Pandemics are extremely serious because the virus can spread rapidly to virtually every country. Because the virus is spread by coughing or sneezing, it is easily infectious, but also avoidable. However, some people infected with viruses can be asymptomatic (have no symptoms, much like the ducks mentioned above), and thus provide no warning. In addition, those that have the virus become contagious before they get symptoms, again spreading the virus without warning. Most people who develop the H5N1 flu have no symptoms from 2-17 days, longer than with most viruses. With our global transportation scenario the virus can thus easily multiply before anyone realizes it and infect a large number of people.

How severe the disease may become and how many deaths it will cause is not known. We do know that in past pandemics, 25-35% of the total population was infected. Estimates are that, with mild disease, 2-7 million people could die; with a highly virulent strain, it would be much higher, infecting 10-25% of the world's population with a mortality rate of 30-40%. That could mean half a billion deaths...or worse. Needless to say, that would be a cataclysmic event that would change the course of the world as we know it for decades to come.

Pandemics can also occur more than once. Since they occur rapidly, it is possible for a community to be hit once, infecting a percentage of the population. While that community recovers, the virus spreads elsewhere and infects other communities. Eventually, it can return to the same community and attack again, either with the same virulent strain or, in a worst case scenario, in a newer and more deadly strain. Based on past pandemics, a second wave can spread throughout the world usually within a year.

THE PANIC OF PANDEMICS

Pandemics are bad enough when thousands of people die of an illness, but what makes them even worse is the panic associated with them, causing even more harm.

How many times have we read about hundreds of people being trampled to death at a soccer match or some huge religious gathering overseas? Almost every year some event occurs in which a panic causes untold deaths. In these cases, a rumor or thoughts of impending problems cause people to act irrationally and without thinking. It is this 'panic mentality' that causes even greater devastation during a pandemic.

One hint of what might occur in a modern day flu pandemic is what occurred with the SARS virus in Hong Kong (see Chapter 1). Once this virus began spreading, it caused more than death...it caused panic. In Hong Kong, a boy falsely declared that an island-wide quarantine was about to be enforced. Many people rushed to stock up on food and supplies, thus depleting those stores in a matter of hours, making those who had not stocked up, or who could not afford to do so, even more concerned. School classes were canceled for two months. Ninety per-cent of the residents wore surgical masks and seventy percent avoided hospitals and medical clinics.

The emotional toll was great. In a study done after SARS, it was noted that over 65% of people felt helpless, horrified and apprehensive because of SARS and 48.4% of respondents perceived that their mental health had severely or moderately deteriorated because of the SARS epidemic. Almost 7% of respondents had psychosomatic symptoms such as sweating, nausea, trouble breathing, or pounding heartbeats when just thinking about the SARS epidemic. When the situations before or during the SARS epidemic were compared, 4.2% of people had family members in need of psychological or psychiatric services, 6.1% reported decreased sexual functions, 37.2% reported a poorer social life, 20.1% of those employed reported difficulty in concentrating on their work, and 26.5% of respondents reported poorer emotional states of their family members.

As a result of these reactions, the inhabitants of Hong Kong suffered far more than from the actual virus itself and we can assume that an avian flu pandemic would manifest itself in a similar manner.

WHAT CAUSES PANIC AND HOW CAN WE AVOID IT?

Panic occurs when people resort to extreme measures to protect their interests. This behavior occurs when, whether realistic or not, it is perceived that time is of the essence and that if you're not expedient enough, your physical survival may be compromised.

In such panic, people may make 'a mountain out of a molehill.' What may not be a real threat becomes an end-of-the-world scenario. This is because the human mind is better at perceiving patterns than analyzing its components. A good analogy can be seen in a series of dots that are laid down in a straight line. Most people perceive that the dots form a line, although a true 'line' is one that is unbroken. The human mind, seeing dots, instantly connects them, creating the impression that there exists a line. Applied to SARS or any viral pandemic, once you see cases spreading, you instantly perceive a broad trend; i.e., it will continue to spread and infect. While this can be the case, it is not a foregone conclusion in the least.

The extent of a panicked public reaction depends on knowledge and information; the less you have of these two, the more panic will ensue. Alarm also increases when you feel the events around you are out of your control. Both of these factors can play a huge role in how people react in a pandemic.

Interestingly, in the SARS reaction above, more than 90% believed that public health measures were an effective means of prevention. Even so, many people still panicked. What would happen if the public does not believe that the government and local officials are prepared? What would happen if the government really wasn't prepared and people found out? The simple answer: pandemonium.

The SARS virus pales in comparison to a possible pandemic from the H5N1 virus. The number of people who could become infected and the number of deaths that would result are nightmarish in the least. And as you will see in the following pages, our local, state and federal governments are not yet prepared for a viral pandemic, especially one as potent as the bird flu. And we, as a people, are even less prepared.

It will be extremely important for our governing bodies to communicate the actual facts of a pandemic, what they are doing to control it, and how people can do their part. If they are not prepared to do so, and we are not prepared to listen and understand and take our own precautionary actions, the consequences are that even more damage could result from the *reaction* to a pandemic than from the actual pandemic itself.

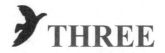

THREE

POSSIBLE SCENARIOS

SCENARIOS OF THE BIRD FLU: HOW IT MAY UNFOLD

There is a lot of conjecture about what will happen with the bird flu, ranging from nothing, to destroying the world as we know it. Obviously, if it becomes contagious among humans, it can certainly cause a pandemic, which would wreak havoc on our country and the world. However, it may never become that virulent or may cause only minor harm.

The following are six different scenarios of what the bird flu has the capability of doing, depending on various factors such as how it mutates, how it spreads, where it spreads, as well as human reaction to its spread. These scenarios will give you an idea of what may occur in the near future, or, what future bird viruses may do in general. Please keep in mind that these are possible scenarios that are based on best-guesses.

From best to worst case:

SCENARIO 0:

Several outbreaks of the bird flu occur in localized regions of the world. The virus is found in chickens and those flocks are slaughtered to prevent the spread. For several years, the virus appears in new regions, but is limited to those regions.

Miraculously, and for unknown reasons, the virus seems to disappear. No new infections are found in chickens, and farmers and ranchers throughout the world relax.

Suddenly, just a few months after the virus disappears, it reappears, both in the same region and some new areas of the world. More chickens are infected and some migratory birds are found dead.

For the first time, the virus is transmitted to humans directly from infected birds. On rare occasions is the virus transmitted from an infected human to someone else, but never beyond that. The virus is virulent and causes death in half the people infected (and 100% of the chickens). Approximately 200 people die of the infection.

Once again, the virus disappears. Whether it is hibernating and will reappear, or has mutated into a non-virulent strain, no one knows.

SCENARIO 1:

Several outbreaks of the bird flu occur in localized regions of the world. The virus is found in chickens and those flocks are slaughtered to prevent the spread. For several years, the virus appears in new regions, but is limited to those regions.

Despite measures to isolate the virus and harvest infected fowl and migratory birds, the virus continues to spread. Fowl to human transmission occurs, but infects only those humans who have had direct contact with infected birds. Some human-to-human transmission occurs, primarily among close relatives of those infected by birds, but also some health care workers.

There is a steady increase in cases reported over several more years, infecting several thousand people. Close contacts are given antiviral medications which reduce hospitalization and the death rate. Nevertheless, approximately 1000 people worldwide succumb to the virus, mostly in third-world countries.

Eventually the virus stops spreading, most likely mutating to a less virulent strain. There are no additional human cases documented, though the virus is noted to be endemic in wild ducks and geese.

SCENARIO 2:

Outbreaks of bird flu virus in humans are reported primarily in Asia and Africa. Investigators from the CDC and WHO document that the H5N1 virus has mutated and can now be transmitted among humans, which raises the pandemic meter to Level 4 (see Chapter 2).

Immediately, all travel to and from those countries is restricted to health workers only. The virus has been tested and appears to be a lower virulence than expected, but still destructive. WHO and the CDC reassure the world that this strain should not cause a pandemic. WHO provides antiviral medications to those infected with the virus and experimental vaccines to people exposed to the virus but who have not yet been infected, to prevent further spread.

The travel restrictions prevent further spread of the virus to other countries. Occasional outbreaks are reported in other Asian countries, but they are contained locally.

Within the affected countries, the virus continues to spread in localized regions, but not to as many people as expected. In these regions, clusters of 15-25 people become infected over the course of two week periods. In most of those infected, virus symptoms are moderate, but much worse and longer in duration than the usual seasonal flu viruses. About 20% of the infected people die, mostly the elderly and those with chronic respiratory or heart disease.

In other countries, people are anxious and many buy supplies and masks in anticipation of a worldwide pandemic. Within a few months, however, the virus has been confined to its original locations. Overall, approximately 5000 people have died in the affected countries.

SCENARIO 3:

Outbreaks of a mutated H5N1 bird flu virus are reported in several countries in Asia and Africa, a result of human to human transmission. Soon, clusters in Europe and South America emerge as well, and a few in North America.

At first, clusters are small, affecting only handfuls of people. In the more primitive countries, it spreads further, but not rapidly, and the spread is limited in European countries by isolating the clusters.

The virus is tested and appears to be lower virulence than expected, but still destructive. WHO and the CDC reassure the world that this strain should not cause a pandemic, but the warnings are guarded. WHO provides antiviral medications to those who have been infected and an experimental vaccine to people exposed to the virus but who have not yet been infected, to prevent further spread.

The spread of the virus slows and appears to be contained. Occasional outbreaks are reported in additional areas, but again are limited to small groups.

After several months, additional clusters of people in the same and in several additional regions suddenly become infected with the virus. This strain of H5N1 appears to have gradually adapted to humans and has become more virulent. It has now affected larger clusters of people, from 25-50, over the course of two to four weeks. Fortunately, the clusters are still localized. It is considered a Phase 5 virus, meaning it has substantial risk to become a pandemic.

The virus is fairly virulent and nearly 30% of people infected have died. Antiviral medications help some people, but in several areas the virus has become resistant. People in civilized countries are on guard and many have started taking precautions and storing supplies. They have been reassured by their governments that this particular virus is not yet fully transmissible and should be containable.

After several more months, the virus is contained and has stopped spreading, but has killed approximately 25,000 people worldwide.

SCENARIO 4:

In Asia and Africa, large numbers of people become infected with the H5N1 bird flu virus. Scientists with the CDC and WHO report that this is a highly virulent strain that has mutated and can be transmitted easily among humans. They have declared the start of a pandemic, Phase 6, and have warned people in other countries to be prepared.

Despite civilized countries taking precautions, the virus quickly spreads throughout the world in a few months. In the U.S., it simultaneously begins on the East and West coasts, but soon spreads to the entire country with steadily increasing numbers of people infected. Reports of deaths are already occurring and hundreds of people who are having flu symptoms are being seen in hospitals and clinics. People who think they have been in contact with infected persons are also going to hospitals, and these institutions quickly become overwhelmed. Doctor's offices are being deluged with calls and telephone lines are being jammed.

Numerous rumors abound on the Internet and quickly spread, overstating the numbers of people infected and describing horrific symptoms. The government begins hourly announcements through television and via the Internet on the CDC and NIH websites. These websites and television updates direct people who have symptoms to local hospitals and other health care facilities that have been prepared for such an occurrence and have available medications and facilities to care for the sick. People who have had contact with infected humans are directed to previously designated local health clinics to receive vaccines and necessary supplies, such as masks, to ward off continued spread of the virus.

All media outlets carry CDC messages at all times and intermittent news updates are broadcast based on CDC bulletins. People are advised to stay home and avoid crowded areas. They are told what to do to protect themselves and their families. They are told to contact their workplace and to stay home if possible. School closings are announced, but parents can go online to obtain homework assignments.

Nevertheless, there is some panic. Grocery stores and drugstores are overrun and sell out of most food, water, and other supplies within days. Fortunately, the local authorities have posted the location of facilities, such as armories, arenas and stadiums, where people can obtain necessary food and water. There are also specific phone lines dedicated to answering questions and directing people to the nearest facilities. People are instructed to wear masks when going to these facilities, or receive them as soon as they arrive.

Doctors, nurses, emergency personnel and firefighters are all coordinated to provide health care to the sick and to those who have been in close contact with those infected. All personnel have received vaccine and wear N95 masks (see Chapter 6) and latex gloves to prevent infection. People who are the most sick or are most likely to die from the virus are given antiviral medications. Those who have not been infected are urged to go to specific facilities and obtain an experimental vaccine. They are also supplied with masks and latex gloves to be used when in contact with others.

Police and National Guardsmen are placed on high alert, patrolling for looting and controlling any violence from the panic. They are also provided vaccines and supplied with N95 masks to prevent self-infection.

Although there are not enough medications or vaccines to treat everyone, there is enough to slow the pandemic. People who have become infected after having the vaccine or taking antiviral medications appear to have fewer symptoms and most do not require hospitalization.

After four to six weeks, only sporadic cases are being seen. Most people have recovered, but almost 25% who were infected have died. Fortunately, due to preparedness, the infection, panic and the resultant death rate are much lower than might be expected, but still almost one million people die worldwide.

The economy of the United States takes a hit as the stock market plummets, businesses lose trillions of dollars in sales and production, workers lose their jobs and income as the service industry dies overnight, which in turn causes a recession.

SCENARIO 5:

In Asia and Africa, large numbers of people become infected with the H5N1 bird flu virus within only one week. Scientists with the CDC and WHO report that this is a highly virulent strain that has mutated and can be transmitted easily among humans. They have declared the start of a pandemic, Phase 6, and warned people in other countries to be prepared.

Despite civilized countries taking precautions, especially restricting travel, the virus quickly spreads throughout the world. In the U.S., it simultaneously begins on the East and West coasts, but soon spreads to the entire country, with steadily increasing numbers of people infected. Reports of deaths are already occurring and hundreds of people who are having flu symptoms are being seen in hospitals. People who think they have been in contact with infected persons are also going to hospitals, overwhelming them. Doctor's offices are being deluged with calls and telephone lines are being jammed.

> "Many doctors, nurses, emergency personnel, and firefighters try to provide health care to the sick, but many are not working and are trying to fend for themselves and their families."

Numerous rumors abound on the Internet and quickly spread, overstating the numbers of people infected and describing horrific symptoms. The media starts reporting the pandemic, showing scenes of panic and overflowing hospitals. Reports are broadcast with statements from the CDC and White House, but are not well detailed and people do not understand what to do, causing further mayhem.

Traffic is a mess, with tens of thousands of people trying to get away from the big cities. Panic runs rampant. Grocery stores and drugstores are overrun and sell out of most food, water, and other supplies within hours. People do not know where to go or what to do to get supplies. There are no local facilities that have stocked emergency supplies, and the few that have remain locked or have been looted.

Many doctors, nurses, emergency personnel, and firefighters try to provide health care to the sick, but many are not working and are trying to fend for themselves and their families. Health care workers wear surgical masks and latex gloves, but most do not have N95 masks, so are at great risk of being infected. Some have obtained experimental vaccine, but most have not. Many of them become infected and die, or simply walk off the job as a means of self-preservation.

Antiviral medications are not conveniently stored and thus are not available as needed. There is no plan in most localities for storage and distribution of medications and vaccine. Most hospitals wait several days and sometimes more than a week to obtain the medications and vaccines. Most hospitals need ventilators desperately but none are available.

Many people have previously obtained antiviral medications and have started taking them prophylactically to ward off the virus. Unfortunately, this begins the development of resistance to the medications, and those who really need the medications cannot obtain them.

After another week, some antiviral medications finally arrive, but don't seem to be helping. Scientists at the CDC report that the viral strain has become resistant to the antibiotics. Even so, there is only enough for less than five percent of the population. Vaccines have helped some people, but most have been unable to receive them. Even so, the H5N1 strain has mutated and the vaccine cannot prevent the infection, although it does lessen the severity.

There are police and National Guard patrolling the streets intermittently for looting and violence from the panic, but many have abandoned their posts. There continues to be looting and attacks on homes to obtain food and water. Those who did stock up and prepare are under siege by those who did not. Car-jackings are occurring by the thousands as those without transport in infected areas will do anything to save themselves and their families. In many areas, electricity is not available and many phone lines do not function. Gangs of youth are seen throughout the larger cities. It's the haves against the have-nots.

Most people stay home from work. Most companies providing food services are closed. In most areas of the country, schools are closed. Many children continue to play outdoors, with nothing else to do.

After many weeks, only sporadic cases are being seen, although clusters of infected people are still being reported.

Many people have recovered, but almost 40% who were infected have died, totaling in the hundreds of millions worldwide. Many of these people were elderly and had chronic disease, but a large percentage were children and young adults. Funeral homes are overwhelmed and thousands of bodies are stacked or are cremated to make room. Funerals weren't held to prevent further spread of the virus.

After several months, the virus has finally hibernated, believed to have mutated into a non-virulent form. Left behind is a world in political, social and economic shambles from which it will take decades to recover.

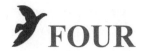 **FOUR**

THE INFLUENZA OF 1918

The avian flu currently making its way around the globe and the avian flu that caused a devastating pandemic in 1918 are alarmingly similar. Examining and understanding what occurred during the 1918 pandemic can provide essential information that can help protect us should the current flu virus spread globally.

There has been ample discussion about what's known as the Great Influenza Pandemic of 1918. There have been comparisons made and lots of misinformation spread about the cause and effect of what happened over 80 years ago that resulted in 50 million deaths worldwide. 16,000,000 people died in India alone, and 650,000 perished in the United States. In the span of 10 months, ten times more Americans died as a result of this avian influenza than the total number of casualties suffered by U.S. servicemen in World War I. None of the more famous infectious agents (Black Death, AIDS, Ebola, SARS, anthrax) have come close to matching the lethality of the 1918 pandemic.

Because of the threat of H5N1, or other avian viruses, becoming a pandemic, researchers have investigated the 1918 virus to help combat the potential spread and lethality of such viruses. In 1996, Doctors Jeffrey Taubenberger and Anne Reid, both researchers at the Armed Forces Institute of Pathology in Washington, D.C., were able to sequence the genetic structure of the 1918 influenza virus. They found that the pandemic was caused by an H1N1 avian flu strain that eventually mutated, enabling human to human transmission.

The H5N1 strain distinguishes itself from H1N1 in that

it has yet to adapt to humans. The unfolding of the pandemic of 1918 illustrates however, that this can change at any time.

> **The flu that hit Haskell County and then 'disap-peared' wasn't dead, just "shocked."**

The fact that H1N1 developed the capacity to spread to humans was an accident of nature. Like the H5N1 virus, H1N1 was Type A influenza, meaning it could only efficiently spread between birds. Other mammals, such as pigs, could pick up the infection as well, and return it back to birds, but not efficiently, meaning it could not spread in a sustained manner. Only by adapting to humans by mutation or sharing information with another virus found in the host could it become more effective and spread sustainably. The former is apparently what occurred.

John M. Barry, historian and author of The Great Influenza: The Epic Story of the Deadliest Plague in History, calls this process "passage" and credits the phenomenon with creating and spreading the lethal version of H1N1. Mutations increased the virus' capacity to adapt and survive in a host that should have been immune to such an invasion.

The first human outbreak of the H1N1 influenza is widely agreed to have occurred in 1918 in Haskell County, Kansas. The area was largely farmland. Contact with fowl and swine was commonplace, creating conditions conducive to contracting bird flu– conditions that may invoke images of present day Asia where chickens and ducks can even be found roosting in human sleeping quarters.

In February 1918, a Haskell County doctor named Loring Miner became alarmed by the number of acute cases of the flu he was seeing and by how healthy those infected had been. "The strongest, healthiest -- the most robust people in the county were being struck down as if they had been shot." [i] Equally as baffling, the outbreaks stopped as quickly and mysteriously as they had started. Schools reopened. People went back to work. The county resumed normal functions.

Dr. Miner, however, could not dismiss the outbreak. He felt compelled to report it to Public Health Reports, a journal dedicated to communicable disease. He warned of "influenza of the most severe type."

The sudden disappearance of the flu in Haskell County illustrates a stage in the life cycle of some mutating viruses. According to Barry, "When the 1918 virus jumped from animals to people and began to spread it may have suffered a shock of its own as it adapted to a new species. Although it always retains hints of virulence, this shock may well have weakened it, making it relatively mild." [ii]

The flu that hit Haskell County and then 'disappeared' wasn't dead, just "shocked." Perhaps it could have run its course and vanished in rural Kansas; the county was both isolated and sparsely populated. And in fact, the virus might have contained itself in any other year. But this was 1918, and there was a war going on.

Young men from all over the country, 56,000 of them, reported to military training at Camp Funston, Kansas. Among them were boys from Haskell County. The barracks were overcrowded and lacked proper heating, prime conditions to spread contagion. On March 4, one of the camp's cooks came down with a fever of 103 degrees. In a matter of weeks, thousands of soldiers on the base required hospitalization or treatment at infirmaries for the flu. Of those cases, 46 proved fatal. The cause of death was ruled "pneumonia."

Again the outbreaks subsided and seemed to disappear. In reality, however, now it was recharging; still incubating, but in far less virulent form. During this time, the 89th Division from Camp Funston was deployed to France, stopping first in England. There the Division received a handwritten message from King George welcoming the Americans on behalf of the British Isles. Scribbled on official stationary was the ironic message: "The Allies will gain new heart and spirit in your company. I wish I could shake the hand of each of you!" [iii]

In April 1918, Nobel Prize winning epidemiologist Macfarlane Burnet noted that "a new strain [of influenza has been established]...The ancestral virus responsible for the spring epidemics in the United States passaged and mutated...The process continued in France." [iv]

The more people the virus infected, the more suited it became to take a deadly turn. Momentum was on its side. By August, pockets of lethal influenza were spattered around the globe: Sierra Leone, Tahiti, Switzerland, India. In September, the virus was at the peak of virulence when it crept back into the United States.

That month, Dr. Victor Vaughan, Surgeon General of the Army, was sent an urgent message to report to Camp Devens outside Boston. Sixty-three men had died there that day. Their autopsies revealed swollen lungs that oozed with fluid and had turned blue.[v] Doctors concluded that influenza was the cause of death. This strain, however, would redefine what it meant to have "the flu."

"Everybody had a preconception of what the flu was. It's a miserable cold and after a few days you're up and around," says Dr. Alfred Crosby, author of *America's Forgotten Pandemic*.

"This was a flu that put people into bed as if they'd been hit with a 2x4. That turned into pneumonia. That turned people blue and black and killed them. It was a flu out of some sort of a horror story." [vi]

From Boston, the flu spread down the eastern seaboard.

Officials of major metropolitan areas either failed to recognize the threat of influenza or brazenly opted to downplay its severity (a reaction not unimaginable today). Philadelphia's public health director, Wilmer Krusen, was guilty of the latter. He went on record to deny that influenza posed any threat to the city. He chose to ignore health officials who advised him to quarantine the Navy Yard that had suffered a major outbreak. [vii] To Krusen's way of thinking such measures would cause panic in the population; in turn, the war effort would suffer. Keeping public morale high took precedence over the health of his constituency.

Philadelphia had organized an enormous Liberty Loan parade that would sell millions of dollars in war bonds. Krusen was urged to cancel it. Health experts warned reporters of the danger posed by the massive public event, but newspaper editors ignored them. They would not disseminate information that could distract from the war effort. The parade went on as planned. Thousands marched as hundreds of thousands watched, all breathing air contaminated with deadly influenza particles.

"One cannot look at the influenza pandemic without understanding the context…These were unusual times. The Great War made them so," explains John M. Barry.

Dr. Alfred Crosby agrees: "There were two enormously important things going on at once and they were at right angles to each other. One was the influenza epidemic which dictated that you should shut everything down, and the war which demanded that everything should speed up. You should continue to have bond drives, soldiers should be put on boats and sent off to France…It [was] as if the country could handle only one big idea at a time and the big idea was the war." [viii]

Within forty-eight hours of the Liberty Loan parade, the flu assailed Philadelphia. Krusen was forced to concede that "The epidemic [was] now present in the civilian population and is… the type found in naval stations and cantonments." [ix]

The disease moved into small towns around the country. Containment was impossible. People tried to protect themselves by wearing masks that proved useless against the microscopic virus. "It was like trying to keep out dust with chicken wire." The epidemic had become a national crisis. Hospitals teemed with the afflicted. There was a severe shortage of doctors and nurses since most had been shipped to aid soldiers in Europe. Those who remained were overwhelmed. The number of patients needing their care was incomprehensible and many came down with the disease themselves.

One army physician, Dr. Roy Grist, wrote a colleague describing the horror he witnessed:

"We have lost an outrageous number of Nurses and Drs...It takes special trains to carry away the dead. For several days there were no coffins and the bodies piled up something fierce...It beats any sight they ever had in France after a battle. An extra long barracks has been vacated for the use of the Morgue, and it would make any man sit up and take notice to walk down the long lines of dead soldiers all dress and laid out in double rows..." [xi]

Victims were ravaged in the process of being killed by the flu. The disease caused extremely high fever that led to delirium. Hospital beds were saturated with blood, sputum, urine and feces. Noses and ears bled profusely. Lungs filled with fluid, drowning the afflicted. Oxygen could not be carried through the body, which turned victims dark blue, almost black, causing some to fear that the Bubonic Plague - "Black Death" - was responsible.

Notably, the age bracket with the highest mortality rate during the pandemic were 20 to 30 year olds- people in prime physical condition. Part of the reason was due to the war. Troops were crowded into ships, barracks and cantonments where the disease spread rapidly. There is no question that this exacerbated the infection rate of young people. However, even if there were not a war, the statistic would likely be the same. It wasn't just soldiers who died, but also pregnant women and children. The flu virus was the type that lent itself to killing those with the strongest immune systems. These young peoples' defense mechanisms overreacted, clogging the lungs and preventing oxygen from reaching the body's tissues.

The pandemic exposed the need for a stronger and expanded federal role in safeguarding the nation's health. Government officials on the state and local levels closed schools, churches, saloons, theaters, auditoriums and anywhere else people assembled. Laws were passed requiring people to wear masks and enforcing anti-spitting ordinances. [xii] "The present epidemic has demonstrated," according to the Surgeon General at the time, "the imperative need of a permanent organization, within the Public Health Service, available with each emergency."

In October, a researcher in Massachusetts discovered what was thought to be a promising vaccine. Cities clamored to receive shipments of the serum. Thousands of people lined up to inoculate themselves, an effort that would prove to be for naught. The vaccine was made with bacteria, which could not protect against a virus. Unfortunately, in 1918, viruses were not known to exist, so no effective vaccine could be developed.

Interestingly, many people turned to alternative medicine to treat what conventional medicine could not. Influenza patients treated osteopathically during 1917-1918 had a 0.025% mortality rate, as compared to the national average of 6% (and 10% for pneumonia patients, compared with 33% to 75% for the national average). [xiii]

On November 11, 1918, the Great War ended. At the same time the deadly influenza had begun to disappear.

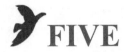

FIVE

DIAGNOSIS AND TREATMENT

DIAGNOSIS: HOW TO KNOW WHEN YOU HAVE THE BIRD FLU

The common (seasonal) flu makes you feel miserable, but how do you know it's really the flu and not a cold? And how do you know if it's a bird flu?

To begin with, both a "cold" and the "flu" are viral infections that cause similar symptoms, such as coughing (bronchial constriction) and sore throat. But, a "cold" is only a minor viral infection of the nose and throat, while the flu is usually more severe, with symptoms that include the sudden onset of high fever and the addition of aches and pains. The fact that flu viruses invade deeper into the lungs and can affect all the body's systems is the reason for the more dramatic symptoms.

Flu symptoms can vary depending on your age:

FLU SYMPTOMS IN CHILDREN UNDER THE AGE OF 5

- Fever
- Nausea and vomiting
- Sore throat
- Nasal inflammation
- Diarrhea

FLU SYMPTOMS IN MOST ADULTS ANDS CHILDREN OVER AGE 5

- Fever
- Chills/sweats
- Fatigue and weakness
- Sore throat
- Cough
- Muscle and joint pain
- Headache

FLU SYMPTOMS IN ADULTS OVER AGE 50

- Fever higher than 99°F
- Fatigue and weakness
- Nasal obstruction
- Confusion

ADDITIONAL SYMPTOMS SEEN WITH BIRD FLU

- Breathing difficulties
- Seizures
- Conjunctivitis (inflammation of the eye)
- Diarrhea, with or without blood
- Vomiting
- Abdominal pain
- Chest pain
- Bleeding from the nose and gums

Symptoms of bird flu may be very different than symptoms from seasonal viruses, as seen above. Several of the victims do not have respiratory symptoms at all and instead are typified mainly by brain dysfunction. Children infected by the H5N1 virus in Asia had diarrhea and seizures rather than respiratory problems. Many of the adults who were infected developed infection of the eyes, called conjunctivitis. Most however, have symptoms from the lower respiratory tract (lungs) early in the illness, rather than later as in seasonal flus. People are more likely to have breathing difficulties and develop pneumonia. Difficulty in breathing develops approximately five days following the first symptoms. Respiratory distress, a hoarse voice, and a crackling sound upon inhalation are commonly seen. Sputum (phlegm) production is variable and sometimes bloody. Pneumonia is seen in a majority of cases.

In patients infected with the H5N1 virus, deterioration is rapid. In Thailand, the time between onset of illness and the development of acute respiratory distress was roughly six days, with a range of four to thirteen days. In severe cases in Turkey, clinicians have observed respiratory failure three to five days after symptom onset. Bird flu symptoms can also progress very rapidly and cause death sometimes within 48 hours. Another common feature is multi-organ dysfunction, meaning that other organ systems besides the lungs start failing. Commonly, this involves the central nervous system and kidneys. When multiple organs fail, the risk of death increases substantially.

As with any flu virus, there is an incubation period; that is, the time it takes for the virus to "set up shop" before it causes symptoms. Seasonal flu viruses have an incubation period of two to three days, but H5N1 virus incubation can range from two to eight days and can be as long as 17 days. As with most viruses, you can be contagious (spread the virus) several days before you become symptomatic.

DIAGNOSIS

The only sure way to know if the flu is an avian subtype is blood testing. To fight the flu virus, our bodies produce antibodies, which attach to the virus particles and destroy them. Different antibodies are created by our immune systems to fight each particular strain, and these can be detected by blood tests. They are 100% reliable and will tell you if you have the bird flu.

Currently, a biological sensor is being developed that can speed up the diagnosis of viral disease, including bird flu. These sensors can detect several types of viruses in five minutes, versus blood tests that can take 1-3 days. A handheld version is being developed to be used in third world countries.

Recently, doctors determined that x-rays of the lungs can determine the severity of bird flu as well as mortality, and can help in diagnosis. All the patients studied who had bird flu had consolidation in multiple areas of the lung. Consolidations are areas in which fluids abnormally fill the lung spaces, becoming a mass. The more consolidations and the presence of air in the lungs (called pneumothorax), the higher the probability of death. These findings can be used to suspect bird flu before blood tests are done.

HOW TO KNOW IF IT'S A PANDEMIC

The warning signal that a pandemic may be beginning is when flu symptoms occur in clusters of people, closely related in time and place. Of course, average flu viruses can spread in clusters as well, so there has to be additional information that this is a bird flu. It can be suspected if it causes more harm (and death) very quickly and is similar to already documented cases of bird flu, then confirmed by blood tests described earlier.

Certainly if these clusters occur in people who have been in contact with chickens or other fowl, it is suggestive that the bird itself may be the culprit. However, if it is spread without the tell-tale signs of the involvement of livestock or fowl, it can be surmised that human to human transmission is to blame, which makes it that much more worrisome.

When clusters of flu are noted, especially in people who have contact with birds, surveillance teams from WHO or the CDC investigate and test those infected to determine what virus strain is causing the symptoms. Of course, this can be handled if there are relatively few clusters. Once there are multiple clusters throughout the world, testing will be limited. However, by that time, we'll know it's a pandemic.

Most likely, a pandemic will start in a third world country, since such countries lack the sophistication to detect and control outbreaks of bird flu before it spreads. Such an outbreak would be devastating to that country since it will not have the ability to deal with a pandemic. It will however, be an early-warning signal for the rest of the world to accelerate their preparations.

TREATMENT OF THE BIRD FLU

So what if you do have the bird flu? How can you treat it and kill it before it kills you?

To begin with, not all people who get infected will die of the bird flu. In fact, the majority will be able to fight the virus with their body's defense mechanisms. You may be very sick, but you'll survive. Most people who survive such a severe strain of flu have no permanent physical damage, although it can worsen pre-existing kidney or liver disease and can cause chronic sinusitis or bronchitis. Psychological damage may linger however (as mentioned in Chapter 2). The main goals of treatment are to prevent the virus from spreading and to prevent death.

It is not known who will survive and who won't. Studies have been conducted for decades in an effort to determine how the virus becomes powerful (virulent), how it wreaks havoc and why some people are more affected than others. So far, scientists have not been able to put all the pieces together in determining what makes the virus tick, let alone how it can be cured or prevented.

The major weapon in today's medical arsenal is antiviral medication. The first two developed were amantidine and rimantidine. Both medications are active against Influenza A viruses, which include the bird flu. These drugs target the matrix protein as outlined in Figure 2 in Chapter 1. By interfering with this matrix, the hemagglutinin protein is unable to gain entry into the cell.

The problem with these medications is that viruses develop resistance to them. In basic terms, the hemagglutinin gene mutates, preventing the antiviral agents from interfering with the function of the protein thus allowing it to enter the cell and replicate. As a result, these medications don't work well against bird flu particles.

Another type of antiviral medication is designed to interfere with the neuraminidase protein instead of the hemagglutinin protein (they are called NAIs, or neuraminidase inhibitors). The neuraminidase protein has an important role in transmitting the flu virus through the body, so preventing this role can help prevent the spread of the virus.

There are two such antiviral medications, Tamiflu (oseltamivir) and Relenza (zanamivir). Tamiflu is taken in pill form and Relenza is inhaled. Both have been shown to reduce the severity and duration of flu virus infections.

Unfortunately, these medications may not be that useful for the bird flu. First, if you don't take them within 48 hours of symptom onset, they won't help at all. Second, and most importantly, these medications don't cure the flu, they just help stem the internal multiplication. Thus it only helps decrease severity and duration. In addition, as Dr. Jeffrey Taubenberger of the AFIP states, "It is quite likely that much higher doses and/or longer treatment courses would be needed to be effective." In most cases, with a seasonal flu virus, these meds decrease the duration by about two days and decrease hospitalization and death rates to a mild degree. However, most flu viruses are not as virulent as a pandemic-creating bird flu virus and so these medications may not be as effective against H5N1.

Another problem with these medications is, again, resistance to the drug. It is one thing if the success rates are modest and quite something else if they don't work at all. In fact, doctors in Vietnam have already found strains of H5N1 that have become resistant to oseltamivir (Tamiflu) in three humans, all of whom died.

Fortunately, in other areas of the world, H5N1 has been found susceptible to these medications, however in 2004, in Thailand, more than three dozen tigers were infected by H5N1 contaminated chicken (there was some thinking that some of the infected tigers transmitted the disease to other tigers) and were subsequently given huge doses of Tamiflu—all the animals died. This caused the CDC to state, in relation to the effects of Tamiflu on these tigers: "Administration of oseltamivir therapy could suppress and prolong the incubation period of the H5N1 virus infection, but it is unlikely."

The bottom line is that these strains of flu, especially the more virulent ones, may develop resistance to these medications. Most scientists and doctors who are being asked about these medications say they should be able to control the bird flu with these medications. They base this on studies of the resistant H5N1 strains, which appear to be less virulent. However, as Dr. Taubenberger says, "Of concern, however, is that no studies have been done on mass usage of NAIs during such an outbreak and whether that could drive the virus to mutate in a way making it resistant but still virulent."

In addition, what if the H5N1 virus mutates into a form

that attacks the nervous system (neurotropic) or the entire body
(pantropic), rather than just the respiratory tract (pneumotropic)? We do not know if these medications would be beneficial
for the treatment of such mutations since they have never been
mass tested on those forms.

When resistance to a medication occurs, it is because
the virus has changed. This change may not only transfer to the
same strain of viruses, but to other strains as well. The problem
is compounded by doctors prescribing (usually on the demands
of their patients) these antivirals for other strains of influenza.
The more people who take these medications, the faster the
strains become resistant. People also may take the medication
when they have colds, not the flu, which again contributes to the
development of resistance.

Another problem regarding treatment has to do with the
amount of medication available. At present, WHO has available
3 million courses (defined as a five day, twice a day regimen),
and the U.S. government has 20 million courses with intentions
to get to 80 million courses, however the current course size
may need to be doubled for an H5N1 strain. Thus, not all Americans could obtain a course of treatment.

So, who will be the first to get these courses? Who
should be the first to get them? They aren't necessarily the same
people.

Certainly health care givers and first responders would
need them because they will be needed to control the virus
and transport and care for those infected. How about everyone
else? The answer would be to give it to those most likely to die
from the infection. But who will that be? With seasonal viruses
(H3N2), the elderly (over age 65), pregnant women, those with
respiratory diseases and other chronic diseases, and care givers, are high on the list. Many authorities have already said that
those are the people who would be a priority. Yet, in the 1918

avian flu, it was healthy adults (ages 20-40) and pregnant women who were most likely to succumb. So the people that need to be protected most may be ones left unprotected. So, which group will most need the medications? As Dr. Fauci of NIAID says, "We just won't know until the virus occurs."

And what about social stratification? Do you have health insurance? Do you have a doctor? Do you feel confident your doctor will prescribe one of the antivirals for you if you ask? Will your doctor remain practicing in the event of a bird flu pandemic? It is not unreasonable to assume that society's 'haves' will find procuring these medicines much simpler than will the 'have-nots', and certainly that is no way to determine who gets the vaccines and who doesn't.

Many governments are stockpiling these medications in case of a pandemic. But spending so much time, effort and money on these stockpiles will be in vain if resistance builds up. As mentioned, in a pandemic there is likelihood that the H5N1 strain would develop resistance. Dr. Fauci goes on to say that "You must stockpile the best you have available and develop new medications in the meantime." In other words, it's the best we have, but we certainly can't rely on it.

VACCINES FOR INFLUENZA

A vaccine is a substance that bestows immunity from specific viruses. In other words, it protects you and prevents you from becoming infected from a particular virus even if you are inundated by virus particles.

Vaccines are designed to replicate parts of the actual virus. These viral portions are then given to a person in a dose or form that won't give them the disease, but will initiate the production of antibodies that can basically handle and destroy those replicated parts and thus wipe out the virus. So, when the person is exposed to the same virus, your immune system "recognizes" these virus parts and immediately sends antibodies to destroy them before they can cause disease. It's as if the school bully had a weakling clone that came to fight you before the bully did, and showed you all his tricks. Having learned the clone's tricks, and therefore the tricks of the bully, (and you've called in all your friends and family to help out), you have a much better chance of besting the bully.

> **Over half the people who die of the flu die from bacterial pneumonia.**

There have been numerous successful vaccines developed, such as the Salk vaccine for polio and another vaccine for smallpox. Vaccines have been developed for types of bacterial pneumonia, for whooping cough (pertussis) and many other infectious diseases. Every year, we have the opportunity to take flu shots, which are vaccines to prevent various flu strains. Even if these vaccines aren't the specific ones and we get the flu, the symptoms are usually milder than those we would otherwise get.

There are problems with vaccines, however. Most are directed against the hemagglutinin spike. With the traditional flu strains, scientists must place their bets on which strain is most likely to spread. The right decision is made only about 50% of the time. In addition, due to mutation, this hemagglutinin protein can change, thus avoiding destruction and/or conferring resistance so that the vaccine won't destroy it.

With the H5N1 strain, scientists know the core proteins already, which is an advantage. In 2005 the US government, through the NIH, isolated an H5N1 virus from a Vietnamese patient. A vaccine was developed from this and early tests show it to be safe and effective against this particular strain. Two problems exist, however.

First, the dose required to provide immunity is much higher than standard doses used with seasonal flu viruses, so much more will have to be made for those who need it. For example, current flu doses are given at 15mcg (micrograms), while this new vaccine has shown progress with doses of 180mcg—a dose 12 times higher. The obvious problem with needing such a high dose is production capacity. Again, this brings to light the problem of not only allocation, but of determination of allocation. Not only who gets it but who decides who gets it.

Second, if the present vaccine becomes ineffective (the virus mutates and changes), another vaccine would need to be made from those infected and would take a long time to produce. In fact, this has already occurred. As of March 2006, researchers have already noted the emergence of a second version of the H5N1 strain. In response, Mike Leavitt, Secretary of the US Department of Health and Human Services, authorized the CDC to begin working on a second vaccine.

The problem is again, what if there are further mutations? If the H5N1 becomes more easily transmissible, it will do so because of another mutation or adaptation. Then yet another vaccine will have to be made. As Dr. Taubenberger of the AFIP relates, "No completely protective vaccine can be made until/unless a particular H5N1 strain emerges as a pandemic because vaccine strains need to match the circulating virus quite closely. Unfortunately, we cannot predict what form of H5N1 will emerge as a pandemic."

These two problems are compounded by time. Simply stated, it takes time to develop and test a specific vaccine. In the most recent case, health officials at CDC and Mike Leavitt had no immediate estimate for the time frame for producing the vaccine. Once the vaccine is ready, then it has to be produced in large amounts, again taking time. It is conceivable that in the first round of the virus, most people would not have access to the vaccine, but would during a second round.

Even so, any vaccine, even partially effective, would be of help. As Dr. Taubenberger points out, "...some H5N1 protection is better than no H5N1 protection." He goes on to say, "What is important about the current process is to work out dosages and adjuvant strategies and conduct efficacy trials to have this worked out in advance of production of the actual pandemic vaccine. Making vaccines using new protocols... are all important to get in place and approved for human use prior to the pandemic."

There is another vaccine, however, that may be of value. Half of the people who die of the flu do so because of a secondary bacterial infection called a 'superinfection.' That is, the virus weakens the respiratory tract and bacteria then invade, with lethal consequences. Over half the people who die of the flu die from bacterial pneumonia. There is a vaccine, pneumovax, to prevent infection from the primary bacteria that causes pneumonia. Currently, pneumovax is recommended for people with chronic respiratory, heart and liver disease and who have no spleen. If a pandemic begins, this vaccine may be able to prevent many deaths from bacterial superinfection.

ALTERNATIVE TREATMENTS: ANOTHER SOLUTION?

Conventional medicine uses medications as their primary tool to fight infectious disease. As I have discussed above, however, these medications and vaccines may not help to any significant degree. Even if they do, there will not be enough for everyone, distribution would be inefficient, and you may be in the low-priority group. So what do you do?

For centuries, people have been using natural methods

to combat disease and have done so successfully. You generally won't hear about these methods however, and no efforts are being made to research them since they are not considered standard medical therapy. That doesn't mean they won't help.

In many instances herbs can be used to treat colds and flu viruses and have had excellent results in comparison to conventional medications. In many cases, the spread of the virus may be prevented or the symptoms derailed, thus decreasing their duration and severity.

These herbs have been discovered to have antiviral properties, so it makes sense they can be effective in combating the flu. What makes them even more interesting is that they have been used for centuries and are still effective, apparently not showing the resistance that conventional medications develop.

Why is this? No one really knows for sure. It is recognized, however, that pharmaceutical companies develop medications typically made of one chemical compound. Herbs, on the other hand, have numerous ingredients that work in concert. It stands to reason that it's easier to develop resistance to one compound than against several working in combination.

Whatever the mechanism, herbs may help significantly in fighting influenza and in a pandemic. Even if you receive antiviral medications, taking these herbs along with them may be more effective than either alone. One thing to remember is that herbs are like any medication in terms of effectiveness. The more often you take them, the less effective they will eventually become, so it's important you take the suggested doses when the need arises, either in a preventative mode when the situation dictates, or when you have symptoms. The following are herbs I recommend to fight flu viruses:

Elderberry

This herb has been shown to reduce the symptoms and

duration of influenza infection when given within 48 hours of initial symptoms. Significant symptom relief seems to occur within two to four days of treatment for most patients, though taking it at the first signs of flu may prevent symptoms from oc-curring. On average, studies show that elderberry extract seems to reduce the duration of symptoms by more than 50%.

Elderberry extract has both antiviral effects and also im-proves immune function. It inhibits hemagglutinin activity and replication of several strains of Influenza A viruses, although it has never been tested on avian flu.

Dosage is 15 mL (1 tablespoon) 4 times daily of elder-berry juice-containing syrup for 3-5 days for adults or a dose of 15 mL (1 tablespoon) twice daily for 3 days for children. In capsules, take 700 mg, 4-6 times per day in divided doses.

Isatis

Isatis (Da Qing Ye/Ban Lan Gen) is a Chinese herb that has been used medicinally since ancient times and is men-tioned in the writings of Galen and Pliny. A constituent of isatis root has been noted to inhibit airway inflammation produced by the influenza virus, according to preliminary research. Other constituents appear to have antiviral, antibacterial, antifungal, analgesic (pain decreasing), and antipyretic (fever decreasing) activity.

Isatis is usually used in combination with other Chinese herbs, the latter of which are designed to improve immune func-tion and increase weak constitutions. Dosage is 1-2 grams daily in divided doses.

Astragalus

Astragalus (Huang Qi) is one of the Chinese herbs often combined with Isatis. Astragalus root has been used to enhance immunity for thousands of years in China and is considered by herbal practitioners to be a tonic that strengthens the body's resistance to disease.

Studies show that it seems to improve the immune response by strengthening the effects of interferon, one of your body's potent fighters against viruses, and by increasing certain antibody levels in nasal secretions. It increases the number of stem cells in bone marrow (that become cells used to combat invading viruses) and speeds their growth into active immune cells. Astragalus also boosts the production of white blood cells called macrophages, whose function is to destroy invading viruses and bacteria.

As soon as you discover the flu, take one 500- milligram capsule of astragalus four times a day until symptoms disappear. Then take one capsule twice a day for seven days to prevent a relapse.

Andrographis

Andrographis is native to Asian countries such as India and Sri Lanka, and is cultivated and naturalized in other areas of the world. Andrographis products have reportedly been used in Scandinavia for more than a decade. One writer credits Andrographis with arresting the 1919 flu epidemic in India, although this has not been proven.

Preliminary evidence suggests that patients with influenza who take a specific Andrographis extract in combination with Siberian ginseng have symptom relief more quickly compared to patients taking amantidine. Patients who take this combination also seem to have reduced risk of post-influenza complication such as sinusitis or bronchitis. It appears to work by increasing antibody activity and phagocytosis by macrophages (cells that destroy invading viruses).

For influenza, a combination of a specific Andrographis extract 178-266 mg plus Siberian ginseng 20-30 mg (Kan Jang) three times daily for 3-5 days has been used. It is standardized to contain 4-5.6 mg of the andrographolide per tablet.

Andrographis should not be used by pregnant women since it may cause miscarriage. This is important since pregnant women are at high risk of complications from bird flu viruses.

Garlic

Garlic is known to kill influenza virus in test tubes and studies have shown antiviral activity against numerous viruses. However, it has not been tested against the avian virus. It also stimulates the immune system and wards off complications such as bronchitis. This herb's aromatic compounds are readily released from the lungs and respiratory tract, putting garlic's active ingredients right where they can be most effective against viruses.

It is recommend that one take several cloves of raw garlic per day during a viral infection, but expose it to the air for at least 10 minutes before consuming, to activate the main ingredient, alliin. You can also take aged garlic extract. Garlic powder or oil may not have the necessary ingredients to fight viruses.

Asian ginseng (eleuthero)

Asian ginseng has immune-enhancing properties, and a protein isolated from unprocessed ginseng root seems to have antiviral activity, according to preliminary research. Ginseng is also widely used as a general tonic or "adaptogen" for fighting the effects of stress on the body, which may be why it may make more potent the virus-fighting ability of antiviral herbs. It is known that taking ginseng for four weeks before taking a flu shot enhances the effects of the vaccine, so ginseng may play a potential role in preventing infection with influenza. There are several varieties of ginseng, including Asian, American and Siberian. Each type appears to have antiviral properties.

Combinations

All of these herbs can be taken together, or can be taken with conventional antiviral medication, which may be advisable considering the H5N1 virus is so virulent. Unfortunately, there are no combinations available that contain all of these herbs, although currently one is being formulated.

WHAT DOESN'T WORK

Lots of other natural products are used to treat flu viruses. Echinacea is the most common herb used for colds and flu because it is reported to have antiviral and immune system stimulatory effects. However, there are no reports that it works against respiratory viruses, which includes the bird flu. Taking echinacea orally might modestly reduce some influenza symptoms but it may also stimulate the immune system. Since many people who die in flu pandemics do so because of overreactive immune systems, echinacea may not be advisable. There is also no standardized form or dosage of echinacea and the products vary widely.

Other herbs commonly used in viral illnesses include vitamin C, zinc, selenium, goldenseal, pau d'arco, larch arabinogalactan, propolis, boneset, and wild indigo. These products are marketed as "immune system supporters" and are usually used alone or in combination with other natural products, such as echinacea. Many other products have less familiar herbs, such as goji, red reishi and humic acid. There is no substantial information that they will work on avian flu, or any other flu, for that matter. Since they are immune boosters, they may also have the same problems as echinacea mentioned above.

Another herb that is being promoted is star anise, which contains shikimic acid, used to produce the antiviral drug Tamiflu. However, huge amounts of shikimic acid are needed to provide antiviral protection and requires chemical modification to make Tamiflu. The bottom line is that you will be wasting your money if you expect any of these herbs to protect you against a bird flu virus.

WHAT TO AVOID

If you are a smoker, you should definitely stop before a pandemic occurs. Smokers are more likely to become infected with flu viruses and suffer more damage to their respiratory tracts. When the lungs are already injured by smoking, it is more difficult to fight off viral infections.

Although alcohol can predispose you to being infected with some viruses, it does more damage by causing you to take higher-risk actions. Because the H5N1 virus is so contagious, having less control of your actions can lead to subsequent contact and infection. Some viruses, especially if combined with others, can cause liver damage, which is another reason to curtail alcohol consumption during a pandemic.

In stressful times, many people increase their smoking and alcohol intake, as was documented during the SARS epidemic. Again, this is not what you should do, since it is likely to result in an increased risk of being infected.

WHAT IS BEING DEVELOPED

At the present time, several scientists from the CDC, the Armed Forces Institute of Pathology, Mount Sinai School of Medicine, and the University of Wisconsin, have been able to extract the bird flu virus that caused the 1918 pandemic. They are attempting to investigate the virus to discover how it works, what makes it virulent, and to possibly find a way to blunt its effects. They may be able to find new medications effective against all viruses or develop a more potent vaccine.

By using a technique called "reverse genetics," scientists can replace any target gene in the 1918 virus with a similar gene from a harmless strain, then measure the effect on the potency of the virus. This allows them to discover the role of each gene. They have already found that the hemagglutinin gene is important for replication and the neuraminidase gene is important for cleaving the cell to help the virus infect it.

These scientists have both the 1918 virus and the current H5N1 virus. Hopefully in the future, they will be able to find out enough about the mechanisms of viral infection to protect future generations from pandemics. Unfortunately, this may take several years or even decades.

Regarding possible vaccines, a British company is developing a universal flu vaccine that would not have to be re-engineered each year. The vaccine would focus on the M2 viral protein, which does not change, rather than the surface hemagglutinin and neuraminidase proteins targeted by traditional vaccines. In addition, this universal vaccine is made through bacterial fermentation technology, which would greatly speed up the rate of production over that possible with culture in chicken eggs (the current method), plus the vaccine could be produced continuously, since its formulation would not change. Still, such a vaccine is years away from full testing, approval, and use. Other researchers are also working on a similar universal agent.

If the H5N1 strain does not become pandemic, it will provide an opportunity to prepare for a future pandemic. As Dr. Jeffery Taubenberger of the AFIP says, "…the ideal outcome would be to use the H5N1 threat to better prepare our pandemic planning, stock pile drugs, work out the technology to make better/cheaper vaccines and increase surveillance. All good things that will be useful when a pandemic does hit."

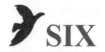 SIX

PREVENTING THE BIRD FLU

The bird flu is here. There is no question about that. When we talk about prevention, there are three aspects:

- Prevent its spread among infected birds
- Prevent a pandemic
- Prevent it from infecting you

PREVENTING THE SPREAD OF H5N1

With bird flu, the first key is to eliminate the birds that contain the virus so it cannot be spread. In all areas of the world where the H5N1 virus has emerged, large numbers of fowl have been destroyed, containing the virus to a specific region.

Millions of chickens have been killed in order to prevent the spread of the virus to other chickens and birds. Nevertheless, the H5N1 virus has spread to other countries and infected other flocks. This has occurred simultaneously, which means that there are factors for spread that are as yet unexplained and thus cannot be controlled.

Most experts believe that the spread is due to infection of migratory birds. We already know that ducks and geese can harbor Influenza A viruses without having any symptoms and numerous reports have documented the death of migratory birds from the H5N1 virus. From Asia, transmission to North America could potentially occur from ducks and geese flying between

Siberia and Alaska. There have already been confirmed cases of H5N1 in Siberia.

In Asia, many people own small flocks of chickens and depend on those flocks for their existence. There are very few precautions they can take to prevent the spread of bird flu in these regions. There is a program by the WHO to vaccinate large populations of birds in countries where the virus has appeared. This may help, but it is difficult to vaccinate tens of millions of birds.

In the US, many chicken farmers are now taking precautions to prevent farm-to- farm spread. They know that such a virus could wipe out everything they own. Visitors are often asked to wash their shoes with water and bleach. Wearing protective boots, masks, and clothing can also help prevent the spread of avian viruses. Most poultry houses are built away from water so as to avoid contact with migratory birds. Most coops are enclosed, which also prevents contact with other birds. Tyson, the largest producer of chicken in the U.S., conducts 15,000 bird flu tests every week to make sure its chickens are not infected.

Nevertheless, the greater risk is of course human transmission of the virus. Even if chickens in the U.S. do not become infected, if chickens in Asia infect humans, the virus will find its way to the United States. So far, human transmission has not continued beyond one person. Humans who have been infected have been isolated or have died, ending the transmission. Only if the H5N1 strain mutates or mixes with another virus within a single host (human or pig) is there a chance of human to human transmission and thus the greatest risk of pandemic. If this occurs, immediate recognition of human clusters of infection will be the only chance to prevent its spread.

Most people who have been infected with the virus are recognized quickly by their symptoms. We do not know if this virus will be able to reside in a human without causing symptoms, meaning that person would become simply a carrier. So far, this has not been identified. However, we do know that the virus is contagious before a person becomes symptomatic and can thus spread the disease before it's diagnosed. This is a more likely scenario.

The World Health Organization hopes to be able to prevent the spread of H5N1 through vigilant surveillance. Their scenario is one in which they start seeing clusters of cases, with the disease extending very quickly…from two to four to fifteen to 20, to 40, to 100 in a short period of time. At that point, a medical SWAT team will be flown to the area, immediately quarantining the site and administering antiviral medications. They hope therefore, to contain the virus to small areas and not allow it to spread. Unfortunately, this depends on a lot of factors, including having doctors able to report these clusters in time and having enough medication to treat effectively. In third world countries, doctors are scarce and medications more so. Officials at WHO worry that if not contained, the virus would spread within a month.

As an extra precaution, people who travel to countries that have confirmed cases should avoid contact with poultry farms and stay away from markets where there are live animals slaughtered or sold. Even coming into contact with surfaces where these fowls have been can cause infection.

In addition, anyone who has developed influenza-type symptoms while overseas in such an area should immediately go to a doctor to be tested. Although standard flu strains are the most likely culprit, it's important to find out for sure.

PREVENTING A PANDEMIC:
ARE WE PREPARED?

Once the flu virus becomes a pandemic, curtailing the

spread is the prime goal, which must be done by the nations of the world. But can that be done?

The World Health Organization and many countries, including the U.S., have decided to stockpile antiviral medications in case of a pandemic. It has been suggested that these medications be used prophylactically, that is, give them to people who are at risk of getting the flu but before they get infected. This would potentially decrease the risk that a fully transmissible virus will emerge or at least it would delay its spread and hopefully provide sufficient time to develop a vaccine.

Unfortunately, this strategy has never been tested and is based on assumptions that cannot be known in advance. One assumption is that the medications will work. Since the major antiviral medication has already been found to be resistant in some H5N1 infected people, the virus may readily become resistant and few people would benefit. Furthermore, in using the medication preventatively, resistance may build up and people who are infected later would not respond to the medication.

The U.S. government currently has 20 million courses (enough for 10 million people if given at twice the usual dosage) but wants 80 million. WHO has only 3 million courses and The Department of Veterans Affairs has 500,000. Even with 80 million courses, many Americans would not be able to obtain the medications.

Furthermore, who would get the medication and vaccines? The Medical and Public Health Preparedness Plan for Pandemic Flu is being prepared by the CDC in order to prioritize just that. At present, plans are to give vaccines to those considered to be at high risk for all influenza; the elderly, those with certain chronic diseases, pregnant women, caretakers, and some children. Yet in the 1918 pandemic, children and young adults (and pregnant women) who were previously healthy were the ones most affected. So this standard policy may not be beneficial for everyone. Medications will be given to those who become infected, but as mentioned, we won't know who is most likely to become infected until it occurs. Thus prompt distribution and delivery will be essential.

This strategy would also require an excellent surveillance program to detect where the virus is and where it is coming from and going to. This would take incredible manpower, especially if the virus spreads quickly, which will most likely be the case. It is quite probable that the virus would always be a step or two ahead of those chasing and tracking it.

To curtail the virus's advance, the authorities would have to restrict access to, and quarantine, areas where it has infected large numbers of people. This again would involve a great amount of manpower.

The question then arises, what if the manpower being used gets infected with the virus? Certainly first responders can protect themselves if they have adequate gear, but how will they know initially that it's a pandemic? There's an increased risk that first responders will also become infected, limiting manpower further.

In addition, in such a pandemic, hospitals would be flooded and would not have the surge capacity to take care of the huge influx of sick people. Most hospitals are privately owned and cannot handle surges of patients as can public or university hospitals. In addition, if medical personnel get infected, a shortage of trained personnel makes things even worse.

Is the world prepared for such a pandemic at this time? The answer is a resounding "NO." Only a small percentage of countries have developed preparedness plans and even fewer have ordered large amounts of antiviral medication. These plans are not in place yet and have never been tested. Is the U.S. prepared? Again, the answer is no. The U.S. is well ahead of other countries, but that doesn't mean it's ready.

The U.S. did create the Strategic National Stockpile after the 9/11 attacks, which contains stores of antibiotics, disinfectants, intravenous hookups and other emergency supplies, which are ready to be delivered to hot-spots within 12 hours. The problem is that antibiotics won't help prevent or treat viral infections and you still need personnel to administer these supplies.

As we saw during Hurricane Katrina, which affected just one region, it is doubtful that we will be able to meet the demands of a pandemic. And make no mistake, a domestic bird flu pandemic would make the Katrina situation look like a skinned knee.

But it does not stop there. Hurricane Katrina showcased other problems. Not only were the local, state and city governments not able to respond adequately, but the federal government followed suit. According to the new plan developed post-Katrina, the federal government will have the primary responsibility for creating stockpiles of vaccines and antivirals, but the states and local governments are responsible for quarantines, delivering the vaccines and antivirals, and getting medical care to those infected. Most states and local governments are totally unprepared.

Most cities will take at least a year to be prepared- or as prepared as possible. Money is also a problem, since local and state governments do not have the funds available or have made arrangements to acquire the funds. Local health departments will receive $350 million from the federal government, but when divided, this provides only $70,000 for each department. That is woefully inadequate. Most states and local governments have limited to zero stockpiles of simple preventive items, such as masks and hand sanitizers, and even less of expensive equipment such as ventilators, each of which cost around $30,000.

Currently, the Centers for Disease Control and Prevention (CDC) are working with local and state authorities to develop their own plans and a general national plan is in the works. However, each state and local government is dependent on their sense of urgency and money, both of which may severely limit the efficiency and eventual success of any plan.

Certainly, if a pandemic occurs, it will be much worse in third-world countries, which do not have the resources to prepare as well as developed nations. As Dr. Jeffery Taubenberger of the AFIP says, "Many parts of the world (where the most people are) will not have ready access to vaccines, antivirals, respirators, or even antibiotics, so may not be much better off than in 1918."

If a pandemic occurs however, even our government may not be able to adequately protect us. Certainly, as time goes by, we can and will become better prepared. As Dr. Fauci of NIAID says, "I think that with each day that goes by we get better and better prepared. We're certainly not where we want to be, but there are activities in place that will get us better prepared."

As well prepared as our government can become, however, we should not solely rely on others. To believe that our government can and will completely protect us is naïve. Therefore, it's up to each of us to take the necessary precautions to protect ourselves and our loved ones.

WHAT YOU CAN DO TO BE PREPARED

If a pandemic occurs, it's incumbent on you to do all you can to be prepared and to prevent becoming infected. Do not rely on the government or anyone else to do so since it is unlikely they can protect you adequately. Realize that, although a person who gets the virus (and survives) may be infectious for a few days to a week, the virus will continue to spread to others for several weeks or even months. So whatever precautions you take will need to last a fairly long period.

The first thing to do is avoid contact with the flu virus. Since the virus is spread through coughing, sneezing and contact with surfaces that contain the virus, you should do all you can to avoid people with flu symptoms and avoid the places where they have been.

To begin with, stay away from crowded areas, especially enclosed areas. Transmission of flu particles is incredibly high in such areas. Certainly this may involve a considerable undertaking. If possible, you might consider traveling to an area that has less of an infection rate. Rural areas would certainly be best, since there are much fewer people and less chance of transmission. Just make sure you are not in the vicinity of farms that possibly have infected birds.

If you are unable to leave your area, if you work with several or numerous other employees, you may have to stay home from work if those infected don't. Hopefully your company will have a policy regarding staying home if you're sick. Having sick people at work, especially with the avian flu, would be the worst thing a company could do, since it's likely that the majority of workers would become infected. Check with your employer or union regarding leave policies and plans for a flu outbreak.

How about your children? Obviously, the flu can spread quickly in schools and your children may have to remain home for an extended period of time. It would be helpful if your children's school had a plan for bird flu. This would entail having assignments for kids that could be done at home or via the Internet. At the very least, you should prepare for your children remaining home-bound for long periods and have materials or things they can do to spend their time constructively.

Obviously, if you can shelter yourself away until the virus passes, you will be better off. However, that isn't always easily done. You also may not have a choice; the authorities may quarantine your area. If you are able to do so, you will need supplies to sustain you during that time. That especially means food and water. If a pandemic hits, everyone is going to be raiding the food stores, and they may be out of supplies or run low very

OTHER SPECIES CAN BE AFFECTED

In early 2006 a cat in Germany died from the H5N1 virus, the first mammal in Europe to be infected. The cat was found on an island in the Baltic Sea, where dozens of wild birds had fallen victim to this virus. It is presumed that the cat ate an infected bird. In Thailand, numerous tigers were found dead of the H5N1 virus also after eating infected birds.

So far, there is no need to worry that these mammals will spread the virus to humans, even though Germany has asked cat owners to keep their pets indoors. There is little risk that humans can be infected from other mammals, other than pigs, which is the only other animal in which re-assortment of viral genes can take place.

quickly. You don't want to spend long hours or even days waiting in line for supplies. Stock supplies and store foods that:

   • Are nonperishable (don't require refrigeration and
     will last a long time); canned and packaged foods,
     dried meats are examples.
   • Are easy to prepare in case you can't cook.
   • Require little/no water (you want to conserve water).

You should consider using a water purifier, either directly on your faucet or in a container, to protect against contamination. Communication is also important so that you can receive information from your local area, so a radio that works on batteries is critical, in case electric lines are not functioning.

Have a can of gasoline stored as well. Gas will be in high demand and there will be long lines of cars waiting to fill up. Hopefully, you'll be prepared enough not to have to travel but be prepared just in case you need to get out of the area to get away from infection.

If you have to go out during a pandemic, you can still protect yourself. Again, however, you need to be prepared well in advance. You should use safety masks so you don't breathe in any potential viral particles. These masks may be in short supply, so be prepared in advance. Most surgical masks and other breathing masks will not protect you against the virus because they allow small particles through. Only the N95 (NIOSH 95) mask can protect you adequately. N95 is a government efficiency rating that means the mask blocks about 95% of particles that are 0.3 microns in size or larger. It meets the CDC guidelines for protection against anthrax spores as well as most foreseeable bioweaponry and avian flu viruses. Anytime you are exposed to the virus, however, you should discard the mask and use a fresh one. It's simply better to avoid other people and exposure.

Another consideration is money. First, it will take money to buy and store supplies, so keep in mind that if you don't have any money saved, or budgeted for such an occurrence, you will be in trouble from the start. Don't rely on ATMs or banks to be open. It's advisable to invest in a safe for your important stores, like cash on hand and your medications, which might be in ultra-high demand come a pandemic.

Additionally, if you take prescription drugs it's very important for you to stockpile at least three months worth. Since many people's lives depend on prescription medications, you don't want to run out and not be able to obtain more.

Finally, understand that in times of pandemic and general panic, lawlessness increases and there will be many people who won't be prepared and will want what you have. For this you must be prepared. One might think this is over-stating the situation, but the fact is that the police will be very much preoccupied with the litany of other issues involved in a pandemic. It is possible that some authorities may even desert their posts to take care of their families. It is because of this that you must be prepared to take your supplies and leave. And as a last resort, if you can't leave, you must be prepared to defend what is yours.

FOODS FOR AN EMERGENCY

If a bird flu virus invades your region, panic will most likely ensue. It won't take long for the grocery stores to be emptied, even by just a few families. As mentioned above, you will want to have enough food stored for at least a month, maybe longer. You also want foods that you can store and that have long shelf lives. In addition, you will want some variety, not only so you don't get bored, but also to balance your nutrients. Here are some suggestions:

Baking mixes
Baking powder
Baking soda
Bay leaves (flour with a bay leaf stored inside the bag)
Beans-dry
Bottled drinks and juices (not refrigerated type)
Bottled water (5 gallon
Brown Sugar
Bullion, concentrated broth
Butter flavoring, Freeze for storage if you can.

CANNED GOODS:

Beans
Broth
Chicken breast
Chili
Diced tomatoes, other tomato products, and sauces
French fried onions for green bean casserole
Fruit
Milk, evaporated milk
Pasta
Pie filling
Pumpkin
Salmon
Soups
Stew
Sweet potatoes
Tuna
Veggies
Powdered lemonade and other powdered fruit drinks
Cheese dips in jars
Cheese soups, like cheddar, broccoli cheese, and jack cheese
Chocolate bars, especially dark chocolate
Chocolate chips
Chocolate syrup, strawberry syrup squeeze bottles
Coffee filters
Corn tortilla mix
Corn meal
Corn starch for thickening
Cream of Wheat
Cream soups
Crisco

DRIED GOODS:

Eggs
Fruit
Onion
Soups
Cocoa
Coffee creamer
Milk powder
Mustard
Noodles
Flour, self rising (if you put bay leaves in the flour, it prevents invasion by insects)
Garlic powder
Granola bars
Hard candy
Honey
Hot chocolate mix
Instant coffee
Instant mashed potatoes
Jarred or canned spaghetti sauce
Jarred peppers
Jellies and Jams
Jerky
Ketchup
Lard
Dry pasta
Marshmallow cream
Marshmallows
Mustard
Table Cream (substitute for sour cream, cream, or half-and-half)
Nuts of all types, try to avoid salted (freeze if you have room)
Pie crust mix plus canned pie filling =cobbler
Oatmeal
Olive oil
Olives, green and black

Onion powder
Packaged bread crumbs
Packaged tuna
Pancake mix, one step, and other mixes that already have the eggs in them
Parmesan
Peanut butter
Pepper
Pickles, relish
Powdered sugar
Power bars
Processed cheese (box)
Raisins
Ravioli
Real butter or favorite margarine (keeps a long time in cool temps)
Rice
Salsa
Salt
Spices and herbs
Dressing mixes
Sugar
Summer sausage
Sweetened condensed milk
Syrups
Tea
Tortilla mix for flour tortillas, wraps, and flatbread
Trail mix
Vienna sausage
Yeast
Baby food, if necessary
Pet food, if necessary

Groceries and other supplies can be contaminated if infected humans have been around those items. If you have food delivered, the foods or the carrier could be contaminated as well. If possible, use disinfectant sprays on such items before storing them and before using them for preparing food.

EMERGENCY SUPPLY LIST

This is a checklist of supplies that you may need in an avian flu emergency. Some of these items you may not need. You will have to determine for yourself which are the most essential:

Gasoline in cars
Water purifier
Safety Masks: look for *NIOSH 95* on the package (see explanation above).
Non-electric can opener
Clorox, plain kind
Dishwashing detergent
Scrub brushes
Paper Towels
Toilet paper
Tissues
Matches
Long-snout type lighters
Candles
Portable heater
Emergency radio
Emergency lighting
Flashlight

Camp stove & fuel
Games, playing cards, crafts
Containers, including at least one 5 gallon or similar bucket (emergency potty and many other uses)
Plastic bags, different sizes, including large ones, many uses
Duct tape
Scissors
Disposable plates, utensils, cups
Cooking pots and a few utensils
Hand beater, non-electric
Ziploc bags
Aluminum foil
Extra set of car keys
Sleeping bags or plenty of blankets
Sturdy shoes
Glasses, sunglasses
Clothes pins
Clothes line rope and other rope
Latex gloves
Work gloves
A little shovel
A small toolkit
Non-electric clock or watch
Batteries
Mylar type emergency blankets
Sunscreen
Alcohol gel hand cleaner
Nail brush
Wipes or baby wipes, refills are usually cheaper (get several kinds, brands smell differently)
Bug repellent, skin type
Insect killers, flying type also
Shaving supplies
Nail clippers

Toothpaste, mouthwash, dental floss
Tampons or other sanitary needs
Shampoo
Soap
No-rinse face wash, like Cetaphil
Mop bucket with wringer to use as a washing machine
Maps, atlas
Metal garbage can to burn trash
Paper and pen
Waterproof marker
Note paper
Photocopies of important documents such as birth certificates, drivers' licenses and so on for the entire family
A *corded* phone, (don't need electricity)
Camping toilet
Generator
Oil lamps and pure lamp oil or propane tanks
Firewood
Kerosene lanterns with fuel & mantels
Items for self protection
Good locks on doors and windows
Water containers
Gasoline containers
Hatchet or Axe
Wound closure strips
Gauze and tape
Band aids
Betadine or Hibiclens to wash injuries
Anesthetic, like Lanacaine or Solarcaine

Vitamins
Imodium (generic is fine and cheaper)
Acetominophen or Ibuprofen
Extra bottles or packages of all prescriptions, B.C. pills
Contact lens solution
Antibiotic ointment
Thermometer
Pet supplies
Camp Stove Indoor-Safe Heaters, Pellet Stoves or other emergency stoves and heaters.

STAY HEALTHY

There are many actions you can take to decrease the chance of being infected, or at least being in good enough health to help fight the infection. These suggestions are good for just general health, but especially important with a bird flu virus.

• Wash your hands frequently with soap and water. Al though viruses are spread by oral secretions (coughing, sneezing), they also are transmitted by hand. If water is scarce (such as in a pandemic), use alcohol-based hand cleaners.

• Keep surfaces clean, especially in the bathroom and kitchen. Again, viruses can harbor on surfaces and you can pick them up easily.

• If you are out of the home, be careful when touching areas that other people touch. Wash your hands if you do. If there is a pandemic, don't be too shy to use latex gloves.

• Cover your mouth and nose when you sneeze or cough and try to convince others to do the same.

• Use tissues and put used ones in a waste basket. Use your upper sleeve if you don't have a tissue.

• Wash your hands after coughing or sneezing. Again use soap and water or alcohol-based cleaner.

• Stay at home and rest if you are sick.

• Eat a balanced diet, especially fresh fruit and vege tables and whole grains. Eat lean meat and fish. Drink lots of water.

• Avoid excess salt, sugar, saturated fat, and alcohol.

• Exercise in moderation, on a regular basis. (If you overdo it you'll tax your immune system and that will make you more susceptible to infection.)

• Avoid shaking hands. The common replacement for shaking hands in areas of viral outbreaks is called the 'elbow bump.' It's all the rage in the infectious disease circles.

COOKING DESTROYS THE VIRUS

Viruses and bacteria are often present in un- cooked or undercooked meat. Whether it is the H5N1 virus in chickens or E. coli in meat or the roundworm Trichonella in pork, cooking will de- stroy these infectious agents. Human infections from H5N1 have occurred from handling uncooked fowl, so washing your hands after handling can also prevent infection.

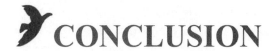

CONCLUSION

BE KNOWLEDGEABLE
BE PREPARED

Having read the previous chapters, you realize that the bird flu is a real and serious threat. You should not close your eyes and pretend it does not exist and that it will not affect you. Even if this particular virus does not cause a pandemic, another bird flu virus eventually will.

The H5N1 virus has not disappeared. It has been present since 1997 and if anything it has continued to spread and become stronger. The longer it persists, the greater the chance it will mutate into a form that can be transmitted among humans. In fact, it has already mutated once, and can do so again at any time.

This bird flu strain is a potent killer. So far, mainly domestic fowl (chickens) and migratory birds have died from the virus, but over half the humans who have been directly infected from fowl have also died, a higher percentage of deaths than any virus yet known to man.

There are anti-viral medications and botanicals that can be used to fight the H5N1 virus, but medications may in fact become ineffective if the virus builds up resistance to them. There are vaccines being developed against the H5N1, but already they have had to be altered due to mutation of the virus. Until an actual pandemic strain is revealed, we won't be able to produce a vaccine that is 100% effective. In addition, due to the potency of the H5N1 virus, much higher doses of medication and vaccine may be required, thus significantly reducing the numbers of people who can obtain them. To complicate matters, we do not even know which people will be more susceptible to infection…and to illness and death.

Our federal government and governments around the world are trying to prepare for the worst case scenario; a worldwide pandemic that will kill millions of people and devastate economies. However, no government is adequately prepared. The more time we have until a pandemic occurs, the more prepared our governing bodies will be, but no one knows when that will be.

At this time therefore, each of us must ourselves be prepared. We must understand what this virus is, what it can do, how it spreads, how it kills and how it may affect our lives. With such knowledge, we can be prepared, thus minimizing the potential for catastrophic damage.

I hope this book has helped you understand and prepare adequately for a viral pandemic. Its purpose is to give you the best foundation for dealing with and surviving such a pandemic. Because this virus is ever changing however, it is important for you to be updated as new developments occur. With that in mind we have developed a website that will contain all the latest information. Log on to www.TheBirdFluPrimer.com, and be prepared.

Larry Altshuler, M.D.

ENDNOTES

i) John M. Barry, The Great Influenza: The Epic Story of the Deadliest Plague in History (New York: Penguin, 2004) p. 89.
ii) Barry, 89
iii) Charles L. Johnston , "Life at Camp Funston: Reflections of Army Sergeant," accessed March 8, 2006, http://members.cox.net/~tjohnston7/ww1hist/
iv) Barry, 180
v) ibid.
vi) "Influenza 1918: Program Transcript," accessed March 8, 2006, http://www.pbs.org/wgbh/amex/influenza/filmmore/transcript/index.html
vii) Barry, 204
x) "Influenza 1918"
xi) Barry, 190
xii Gary Gernhart, "A Forgotten Enemy: PHS's [Public Health Service] Fight Against the 1918 Influenza Pandemic" December 2005, accessed March 8, 2006, http://www.history.navy.mil/library/online/influenza_forgot.htm
xiii) Gilbert E. D'Alonzo, Jr, DO, AOA Editor in Chief, "Influenza Epidemic or Pandemic? Time to Roll Up Sleeves, Vaccinate Patients, and Hone Osteopathic Manipulative Skills" JAOA • Vol 104 • No 9 • September 2004 • 370-371, accessed March 6, 2006, http://www.jaoa.org/cgi/content/full/104/9/370

ACKNOWLEDGEMENTS

I would like to thank my wife Claudia, my daughter, Lindsey, and Rob Shaff for their advice, support and feedback. I appreciate Dr. Jeffrey Taubenberger of the Armed Forces Institute of Pathology and Dr. Anthony Fauci of the National Institute of Allergy and Infectious Disease, and Rich Macary, for providing their time and expertise to contribute to this book. I would further like to thank my publisher, Drew Nederpelt, for his foresight, ideas, suggestions and confidence in my authorship. Thanks also to Lorraine Szypula for her research contributions as well as to Catherine Reinehr and Polina Bartashnik at Sterling & Ross for additional assistance.